Cultural Studies of Science and Medicine

Series editor

Atwood D. Gaines
Case Western Reserve University
Cleveland, OH, USA

More information about this series at http://www.springer.com/series/15110

James Rodger · Zachary Steel

Between Trauma and the Sacred

The Cultural Shaping of Remitting-Relapsing Psychosis in Post-Conflict Timor-Leste

Springer

James Rodger
South Devon Child and Adolescent
Mental Health Service
Devon Integrated Children's Services
Totnes, Devon
UK

Zachary Steel
School of Psychiatry
University of New South Wales
Sydney, NSW
Australia

and

St John of Health Care
Richmond Hospital
North Richmond, NSW
Australia

and

The Black Dog Institute
Randwick, NSW
Australia

Cultural Studies of Science and Medicine
ISBN 978-3-319-24422-8   ISBN 978-3-319-24424-2 (eBook)
DOI 10.1007/978-3-319-24424-2

Library of Congress Control Number: 2015960238

Printed on acid-free paper

This Springer imprint is published by SpringerNature
The registered company is Springer International Publishing AG Switzerland

Very few psychotic episodes last less than 1 month and those that do we know almost nothing about

(Keith and Matthews 1991, 60)

There is one truly serious question in psychiatry, and that is psychogenesis

(Berrios 2003, 9)

Perhaps because the sky becomes dark, so too people's minds become dark

*(*Family member of episodically unwell psychotic person in Timor-Leste*)*

Preface

This work is the result of a long period of reflection, discussion and further reading, following a nine-month period of field work in Timor-Leste in 2004. While ostensibly the study's aims were in keeping with that of conventional and cultural psychiatric epidemiology, in the wake of the countries recently won Independence in 1999 and prior history of colonial violence, we quickly came up against powerful and palpable cultural realities, through which the East Timorese articulated their present and past daily life experience, and which posed a challenge to Western psychiatric epistemology and ontology. For example, in relation to the countries fight for Independence, many people, including in our local team, invoked ideas of magic, as contributing to the resilience of the country's freedom fighters: tree bark tunnelled under the skin was said to render the skin impervious to the bullets of the enemy. We also heard how four sacredly held crocodiles—symbolic creatures of the islands' geographical contours and recounted in creation myths—crawled out of the sea onto a beach in the capital Dili, on the eve of the UN Independence vote, bringing confidence and portending to the people a successful outcome. More closely related to our own work, people spoke of the powerful unseen forces: water and land spirits (Tetum: *bai nain* and *rai nain*), ancestral powers, and sacred houses (Tetum: *uma lulik*) and objects—linked to manifestations of both physical and mental illness. People we spoke with regularly invoked the name of *Maromak*, the Tetum word for God, with tangible feelings of belief, forgiveness and hope, despite the country's troubled history.

Laderman (1994) writes of the anthropologist's embodiment of cultural symbols, and indeed, our experience was that these unseen but felt and spoken realities were compelling, and over a relatively short period of time began, in some way, to feel palpable to those of us out in the field. We were aware that the original terms of reference of our work, based in Western psychiatric nosology, were at odds with the ways of understanding of local people both in relation to trauma and mental illness. While not wishing to downplay the value of previous more epidemiological-based publications from this work, we felt compelled to tell a contrasting (but hopefully complimentary) story about the social and cultural shaping and *containing* of distress, in particular of trauma-related dissociation and psychosis, in Timor-Leste.

However in moving from the supernatural world of Timor-Leste to the secular understanding of anthropology and Western psychiatry–psychology contained herein, we inevitably commit some level of "interpretive violence" (Bibeau and Corin 1995) in reflecting on the nature of such experiences. Prior work and our own study suggests that East Timorese people do dialogue and move between different registers of explanation, according to need and context, and that traditional beliefs and practice can be necessarily resistant to change where serving a useful function. Nonetheless, it was also clear that mental illness and/or distress was a salient concern within Timor-Leste and a problem not wholly solved by local responses, the analysis of which is further complicated by forces of acculturation and socioeconomic change, beyond that of the recent introduction of certain Western mental health concepts. Nonetheless, our aim is not to influence the beliefs and practices of the people of Timor-Leste, but rather we would anticipate our primary audience to be that of Western-trained clinicians and researchers with whom we hope to be able to further contribute to an understanding of cultural patterned distress and disorder, respect for clinical complexity and the psychological "work of culture".

We hope the work will be of value to specialists and students, in both research and clinical work, across the range of disciplines from which we have drawn, including transcultural and critical psychiatry/psychology/psychotherapy, medical anthropology and sociology, critical and cultural neuroscience, psychiatric epidemiology and epistemology, international public health (including the *global mental health* movement), and psychoanalytic and cultural studies.

In preparing the manuscript, we are especially grateful for the inspiration and tolerance of our families and friends, the support and flexibility of the Springer Editorial Team, and the local project workforce, in particular the team manager and assistant manager, who provided cultural consultancy to the project, helped negotiate access with participating communities, and oversaw the data collection process. Cultural consultancy was further supported by the three local interpreters who assisted our study, alongside a separate interview with a traditional healer, and extensive discussion with an East Timorese mental health worker with an additional background in philosophy. Not least we are also indebted to the communities and community leaders of Timor-Leste, who courageously told us their histories of both resilience and distress, and whose accounts inspired the writing of this book. While written in a very different cultural key, we hope that we have done justice to both their courage and their experience.

Note on Identity of Persons Described in Case Material

In order to preserve the anonymity of persons described in case material, names, specific location, *narrow* ethnolinguistic grouping and other sensitive identifying features have been changed or withheld. We hope that we have achieved this with minimal compromise to more essential material necessary for our analysis.

References

Berrios, German E. 2003. Forewords (I). In *Psychogenic Psychoses,* ed. Wimmer, August. *1916* (trans: Johan Schioldann), 9–15. Adelaide, South Australia: Adelaide Academic Press (Original work published 1916).

Bibeau, Gilles, and Ellen E. Corin. 1995. From submission to the text to interpretive violence. In *Beyond textuality: asceticism and violence in anthropological interpretation*, eds. Gilles Bibeau and Ellen E. Corin, 3–54. Berlin: Walter de Gruyter.

Keith, Samuel J., and Susan M. Matthews. 1991. The diagnosis of schizophrenia: A review of onset and duration issues. *Schizophrenia Bulletin* 17(1): 51–68. doi:10.1093/schbul/17.1.51.

Laderman, Carol. 1994. The embodiment of symbols and the acculturation of the anthropologist. In *Embodiment and experience: The existential ground of culture and self*, ed. Thomas J. Csordas, 183–98. Cambridge University Press.

Contents

About the Authors

James Rodger is a Consultant Child and Adolescent Psychiatrist in the UK National Health Service and an Honorary Associate Research Fellow at the University of Exeter. He holds an additional degree in Medical Anthropology and has undertaken postgraduate training in systemic practice. His principle clinical and research interest is the developmental, social and cultural aspects of psychotic phenomena and related implications for intervention. He undertook the key fieldwork forming the basis of this work in 2004, in the context of an 18-month mental health research programme in Timor-Leste. In addition, Dr. Rodger has provided expert evidence relating to transcultural trauma-related psychiatric presentations for both asylum and criminal cases. Previous publications relate to the wider epidemiological research findings and implications from Timor-Leste, to critical-relational challenges to psychiatric practice, and to the anthropology of altered mental states.

Zachary Steel holds the St. John of God Professorial Chair of Trauma and Mental Health, School of Psychiatry, University of New South Wales and Richmond Hospital, New South Wales, Australia. Dr. Steel has developed a programme of mental health research across culturally diverse communities and settings with a particular focus on traumatic stress, forced displacement, conflict and culturally specific symptoms of mental disorder and distress. Within the Asia-Pacific region he is involved in collaborative mental health research programmes in Vietnam, Aceh-Indonesia, and Timor-Leste as well as with asylum seeker and refugee communities in Australia and amongst Aboriginal communities in Far West New South Wales. His research with asylum seeker populations in Australia has helped to develop an evidence based on the adverse mental health consequences of harsh asylum policies including the use of immigration detention and temporary protection visas.

Abbreviations

AOC	Acute-on-chronic
APA	American Psychiatric Association
ATPD	Acute and transient psychotic disorder
BP-	Case history prefix—brief-remitting-relapsing psychotic-cohort
BPD	Brief psychotic disorder
BPNOS	Bipolar disorder not otherwise specified
BRR	Brief-remitting-relapsing
CP-	Case history prefix—acute-on-chronic psychotic exacerbation cohort
DID	Dissociative identity disorder
DSM	Diagnostic and Statistical Manual (of Mental Disorders)
EE	Expressed emotion
FRS	First-rank symptoms
GAF	Global assessment of functioning scale (from DSM-IV)
HTQ	Harvard Trauma Questionnaire
ICD	WHO International Classification of Disease—Mental and Behavioural Disorders
K10	Kessler Psychological Distress Scale
MPD	Multiple personality disorder
OR	Odds ratio
PDNOS	Psychotic disorder not otherwise specified
PTSD	Post-traumatic stress disorder
RR	Relative risk
SCID	Structured Clinical Interview [for DSM-IV-TR]
WHO	World Health Organisation

List of Figures

List of Tables

List of Principle Case Histories

Note
Case histories have the prefix BP- (brief-psychosis) denoting brief-remitting-relapsing psychosis and CP- (chronic psychosis) denoting acute-on-chronic psychosis.
Further direction to commentary on these case histories and to additional briefer case material can be found in the index.

Chapter 1
The Historical, Cultural, Epistemological and Research Context of Remitting-Relapsing Psychosis in Timor-Leste

1.1 Introduction

The island of Timor is a mountainous tropical land formed from the violent opposition of the Australian and Asian tectonic plates and lies at the far southeast of the Indonesian archipelago (Fox 1996). Now divided into Indonesian West Timor, and the more recently sovereign East Timor or Timor-Leste, the occupation and control of the island had long been bitterly contested by Dutch and Portuguese companies trading sandalwood, and later by colonial governments, culminating in a negotiated partition into East and West Timor ratified at The Hague in 1916 (Fox 1996). The more longstanding "indigenous" inhabitants[1] of Timor also bitterly resisted trade exploitation and European colonisation, and it is acknowledged on both Dutch and Portuguese sides that Timor was never pacified (Fox 1996; Gunn 2001). As a Scots sea captain, Alexander Hamilton, writing in 1727 observed, both sides "found that the Timoreans would not lose their liberty for fear of loss of blood" (Hamilton 1930, II:74, cited in Fox 1996).

Ultimately however, West Timor went on to secede less problematically from Dutch control, following the Dutch surrender in the Indonesian War of Independence in 1949, and became part of the new Republik Indonesia Serikat (Farram 2010). In contrast, Indonesian annexation of the vastly more ethnolinguistically diverse Timor-Leste following Portuguese withdrawal in 1975—under the pretext of local self-determination and the need to counter a growing Communist threat—was bitterly opposed by local peoples and resulted in a protracted campaign of guerrilla resistance until independence was finally gained in 1999 (Niner 2001).

[1]Austronesian and later Trans-New Guinean ethnolinguistic groups have long inhabited the island, the former dating back at least 5000 years, and Timor is considered one of the important "gateways for the movement of populations to Australia" (Fox 1996, p. 2).

J. Rodger and Z. Steel, *Between Trauma and the Sacred*,
Cultural Studies of Science and Medicine, DOI 10.1007/978-3-319-24424-2_1

Our study, the East Timor Mental Health Study (conduced February to November 2004) arose out of a perceived need for rich quantitative and qualitative data about the mental health of the Timorese population, in the context of this recently won independence and to support emergent health services (including mental health), in the wake of the atrocities they endured in the protracted fight for this sovereignty (culminating in the widely publicised tragedy following the successful 1999 UN independence referendum).

Following earlier work that appeared to document distressingly high rates (34 %) of Post Traumatic Stress Disorder (PTSD) in the aftermath of 1999 (Modvig et al. 2000), a continued focus on the evolving psychosocial sequelae of trauma remained an important focus of our study. It had been, however, a long established policy of our group to try and reach out and identify sufferers of other mental health problems, beyond PTSD (Silove et al. 2000).

With these goals in mind, and in discussion with government and local health care providers, an epidemiological study was set up in an attempt to quantify and qualify a wide range of mental health concerns, inclusive of, but not limited to "traumatic reactions" drawing on techniques from both traditional and cultural epidemiology, and supplemented by insights from existing ethnography. Such culturally sensitive approaches increase the prospect that differential local experiences, and illness narratives, are acknowledged and recorded vis-à-vis Western universalistic assumptions and illness categories, from which the former may significantly and informatively diverge.

Indeed we report on a significant local pattern of brief but recurrent changes in mental state and behaviour, akin to psychosis, frequently described to us. While such episodes were often triggered by the kinds of family and social stressors that would be familiar to Western mental health professionals, they were also commonly described to coincide with the presence of the new/crescent moon (Tetum: *fulan lotuk*—literally "slim moon") and at other times of cultural significance. Alongside this unfamiliar and unexpected presentation, we encountered comparatively low rates of PTSD and chronic psychosis (schizophrenia and bipolar disorder; see Sect. 1.6, Footnote 17). Interpretation of these key findings, and the tentative relationship between them, forms the focus of this work. In particular, in linking such presentations with tacit histories of trauma and loss, embedded in local cosmological beliefs and networks of meaning, and enacted in specific social contexts, we propose that the recurrent brief-psychotic states documented here, may represent a culturally patterned, and socially mediated alternative response to loss, trauma and adversity.

Linking trauma with brief psychotic experience connects to both the rich historical literature on reactive/psychogenic psychosis, strongly influenced by Scandinavian psychiatry in the early to mid-20th century (e.g. Faergeman 1963; Wimmer [1916] 2003), but also with contemporary research findings relating both childhood and adult trauma, loss and cumulative adversity to psychosis risk (Morrison et al. 2003; Read et al. 2005). Neither body of work has however seriously engaged with questions of culture and the Scandinavian tradition shared the primitivistic assumptions of the period in relation to non-Western societies.

In exploring these issues and those pertinent to psychological and anthropological understandings of trauma, we position the concept of *dissociation*, as a central construct, bridging individual and sociocultural models (Seligman and Kirmayer 2008), as well as providing a plausible schema for thinking through an emerging understanding of the relationship between trauma and psychosis. At a descriptive level dissociation implies a lack of integration of mental processes and/or self-parts, and therefore the constructs (and arguably experience) of dissociation and psychosis have considerable overlap and indeed historically were not so distinct (Moskowitz 2008; see Sect. 5.1). Dissociative disorders have also long been argued to exhibit significant "cultural pathoplasticity" (Spiegel et al. 2011) and dissociative models therefore may have further relevance to our present ambitions, in understanding the unique cultural temporal-spatial patterning of brief psychotic episodes in Timor-Leste. This premise is further supported by recent work pointing to an impact of culture not just on content but on the very structure of psychotic experience (Luhrmann et al. 2015; McLean et al. 2014).

The concept of dissociation also illustrates the competing epistemologies of psychiatry, namely the unresolved—and according to Littlewood (1996) unresolvable—tension between agentic and deterministic accounts of human experience and behaviour (see Sect. 1.7.2)—the former acknowledging the subject has having an active, motived role (albeit often an unconscious one), the latter treating the individual as a passive object of impersonal forces (whether biological or environmental). Concepts of trauma must straddle this dualism however since while the traumatic event itself may often be largely or wholly externally determined, the impact on the person presupposes a concept of agency—for it is precisely through violation of agency that even primarily physical trauma becomes *psychologically* traumatic.

In thinking about *cultural pathoplasticity*, building on the work of Kirmayer et al. (1994, 1996; Seligman and Kirmayer 2008), we give central place to the role of narrative (see Chap. 4) which we propose as the bridge between anthropological and traumatic models of dissociative-psychotic phenomena (cf. Kirmayer 1994; 1996; Seligman and Kirmayer 2008) but also accommodating both agentic and deterministic understandings. We argue that narrative injury unites conventional bodily trauma with other types of culturally-symbolic or moral injury (although of course both types of injury often co-exist—see Sects. 2.3 and 4.1.2) but against this current, culture—expressed and mediated through narrative or unspoken cultural scripts—can be a key organising principle, able to bring greater order to fragmented/dissociated states of mind, even if superficially such order may be far from apparent (see Sect. 4.2.2).

Turning to a richer account of the relationship between culture and psychosis also brings us into the territory of medical anthropological theorising exploring the relationship between culture and asserted better outcomes of schizophrenia in the so called "developing world" (Jenkins and Barrett 2004; Hopper et al. 2007; Hopper 2008; Myers 2011). In this light our findings in Timor-Leste beg an important question. Could the relatively high rates of brief psychotic presentation and the comparatively low rates of chronic psychotic disorders such as schizophrenia be directly related to features of the sociocultural context in Timor-Leste that limit the transition from brief to chronic disorders? Such a question has been asked within psychiatric epidemiology (Castillo 2006; Stevens 1987) but rarely systemically explored. One difficulty noted in drawing on the wider literature in this area however, is that the cultural assumptions underpinning explanations for the better prognosis of schizophrenia in developing countries, are open to significant criticism for relying on somewhat Romanticized notions of so called traditional culture, rarely evidenced by ethnographic work (Hopper 1991; Lucas and Barrett 1995).[2] We therefore have an opportunity to provide support, as far as our data will allow, for previously speculative ideas in this area, in addition to generating new hypotheses.[3]

Indeed while much of work and theorising about better outcomes of schizophrenia have relevance to an understanding of brief psychosis, few culturally sensitive studies have focused specifically on brief psychotic phenomena. While there is a rich colonial and early post-colonial psychiatric literature describing and theorising atypical, often brief psychotic states, in different non-Western cultural settings, with authoritative and representative works including Jilek and Jilek-Aall's (1970) comprehensive review of "Transient Psychoses in Africans" and Yap's (1967) important work on "culture-bound reactive syndromes," concepts of both culture and psychopathology are now understandably dated in these works. Conversely, in more modern epidemiological studies of brief psychosis, detailed consideration of the sociocultural context, above and beyond crude epidemiological indices, is conspicuously absent. Good's (2004) ethnographic exploration of brief psychotic phenomena in Java is therefore an important exception, which he encourages others to follow, although he leaves the question of the relationship between brief and chronic disorder open for others to address. Guinness' (1992a, b) work is also exceptional, in seeking to explore links between stress, culture and psychosis in a non-Western setting, including a direct exploration of the putative relationship between brief and chronic psychosis, similarly using the concept of dissociation as a bridge. This work might be seen as an early prototype of the kind of analyses we have attempted here. However, Guinness' work was not conducted in a high trauma, post-conflict setting of comparable context and his models of dissociation lack the conceptual clarity afforded by recent work and

[2]Furthermore because the very validity and utility of the schizophrenia concept is itself critically contested, Hopper (2008, 198) further notes the paradoxical tension inherent in attempts to solve the "epidemiological puzzle—elevated rates of schizophrenia…—using the interpretive tools of an anthropology premised upon distinctive 'sociocultural' constructions of psychiatric disorder." While acknowledging the difficulty of this problem, we would argue that the schizophrenia concept can nonetheless be used pragmatically for thinking about the links between brief and more chronically disordered psychotic-states.

[3]Inevitably we will generate more questions than we can answer, but in doing so we hope to provide openings for future research. In tentatively reaching for some answers, we have however drawn upon contemporary research, exploring the impact of a wider range of sociocultural mediators, including novel psychosocial interventions, arguably influencing transition rates from first-episode or brief-psychosis to chronic disorder in different sociocultural contexts (see Sect. 5.2).

cross-disciplinary syntheses. Attention to the childhood developmental dimension of psychotic vulnerability is also absent.

In our own attempt to address the developmental domain we note that in his study of recurrent brief psychosis in Java, Good (2004, 189), again ends with an appeal to "explore developmental issues and primary relationships…for individuals who suffer intermittent psychosis," which he returns to address himself in a later paper (Good 2012), now advocating for a psychoanalytic perspective over his previously favoured cultural phenomenology. He advocates attention to "how primary, developmental attachments and relationships structure an individual's inner life over time, [and] of how these—often unbeknownst to each individual—shape what is experienced as real" (Good 2012, 26). Psychoanalytic perspectives have much to offer in this respect, and there is a rich seam of psychoanalytic interpretive work with psychotic individuals, from the mid to late 20th century to mine for insight (e.g. Jackson and Williams 1994; Lucas 2008; Rosenfeld 2013; Searles 1961)—if we can hold in mind the historical and cultural framing.

Useful psychoanalytic perspectives on psychotic-dissociative phenomena have also made it into the transcultural literature, most notably in the work of Obeyesekere (1984), and although not necessarily shared by all (cf. Desjarlais 2012), there is increasing recognition amongst anthropologists of the limitations of cultural phenomenological (Good 2012; Hollan 2012) and textual interpretive–hermeneutic approaches (Bibeau 1997) when faced with complexities of mental illness. Yet appropriation of psychoanalytic insights by social scentists has also been criticised, not least for its over-reliance on Freud and sometimes Lacan, in apparent ignorance of more contemporary developments (Mizen 2009). In response Hollan (2012) and Lambek (2003) has called for the incorporation of ideas from object–relations theory and *relational psychoanalysis* into medical and social anthropologies, in line with the relational concerns and focus of these disciplines. Relational psychoanalysis itself owes much to the rapprochement between psychoanalysis and *attachment theory*[4]—the latter being a theory par excellence of how early carer-child relationships affect later relational patterns and the ability to integrate and regulate emotional life.

We will argue contemporary attachment theory as having an important place in the developmental understanding of dissociation–psychosis, provided suitably revised in cultural context (cf. Otto and Keller 2014; van IJzendoorn and Sagi-Schwartz 2008; see Sect. 3.2). Attachment theory is given due recognition by some Western theorists of the trauma–psychosis link (Benamer 2010—edited vol.; Giovanni Liotti and Gumley 2008), but is often invoked alongside the work of Pierre Janet rather than Freud since in both attachment theory and Janet's work the

[4]Attachment theory was historically distinct and in competition with psychoanalytic models of mind and behaviour. Although more recently it has influenced contemporary psychoanalytic discourse (Fonagy et al. 2008)—including the development of "relational psychoanalysis" (Mitchell and Aron 1999)—these incorporations have rarely found their way into the works of psychoanalytically orientated anthropology, which generally continues to invoke more dated psychoanalytic models (Hollan 2012; Lambek 2003).

external reality of early relationships is given greater weight than the role of internal phantasy ascribed by Freud and many of his successors.

Only rarely have such differential insights made it into the transcultural psychiatric literature. Castillo's (1994a, b) important work, similarly invokes Janet and critiques Freud in his reappraisal of dissociative–psychotic phenomena from ethnographic examples of spirit possession in South East Asia. In a more recent critical medical anthropological inquiry into witchcraft accusations and idioms of spirit possession in children in Northern Uganda, Reiss (2013) also gives much needed attention to the impact of wider social conflict and adversity on family structure, parenting and parent-child relationships, although conspicuously she did not refer to the literature on *attachment theory* which we believe could have added further conceptual clarity and empirical weight to her analysis (see Sect. 3.2).

We will deal with this tension between internal and external realities at length (see Sects. 3.1.3 and 3.1.4) but the two approaches need not be in conflict. As Good (2012, 26) notes in addressing "complex psychological experiences," such as psychosis, a psychoanalytic perspective on subjectivity can complement a "subjectivity shaped by repressive and hegemonic political and administrative structures, gender ideologies, and histories of violence" and both have clear relevance for our present work. We will also argue for the relevance of contemporary developmental models of self, born from the discipline of infant observation (Fonagy et al. 2002; Gergely and Watson 1999; Holmes 2001), but as with attachment theory, such models require some cultural interrogation and revision (see Sect. 3.2), as indeed acknowledged by one of their key theorists (Stern 2003).

It is important to note that medical anthropologists and transcultural psychiatrists are continuing to ask searching questions of methodologies and epistemologies related to cross-cultural understandings of mental health and ill-health. This relates not just to nuanced understanding of culture and more sophisticated understandings of psychological processes, but moreover identifying a need for multiple levels and domains of analysis and explanation from the biological to the political (Hinton and Kirmayer 2013; de Jong and Reis 2013)—to include developmental dimensions (Kirmayer and Crafa 2014; Reis 2013), which we partly address in our discussion of psychoanalytic and attachment perspectives. It also calls for an exploration of relationships between such domains, recognising that a productive change at one level (e.g. the individual), may be harmful at another level (e.g. societal), with relevance to both aetiology and intervention[5] (Kirmayer 2012).

With this in mind, we go on to explore not only the influence of culture on illness but also the impact of illness (including diagnosis and treatment) on culture.

---

[5]A good example of such analysis include the study already noted, by Reis (2013), looking at the catastrophic individual consequences of witchcraft accusations targeting children in Northern Uganda despite the possible *short-term* group utility of such behaviour (see also Sect. 1.7.3). Also relevant to the present analysis is a range of work looking at the implications for cultural concepts of self, of psychiatric medication uptake (e.g. see special section on "The Anthropology of Psychopharmaceuticals" in *Culture, Medicine and Psychiatry* 2012, 36(1) and Jenkins 2011-edited volume).

In particular we explore the revitalisation of traditional cultural practices and ideas in Timor-Leste, and drawing on contemporary systems and communication theory, we ask what, if any relationship this may have, to the patterns of brief-psychosis, we encountered (see Sect. 4.2.3). Significantly, for our purposes, many of the classical anthropological accounts of religious or cultural revitalization (e.g. Fernandez 1978; Worsley 1987), as well as a more contemporary account from Timor-Leste itself (Traube 2007), describe a charismatic individual articulating a revised cultural vision under the sway of some greater force, which descriptively (from a secular perspective) have a dissociative quality to them.

As should already be apparent, we have tried to bring together a diverse range of literatures for consideration. While there has been fruitful inter-disciplinary dialogue between some of these areas (for example exploring links between trauma theory, dissociation and developmental models of psychosis; and between anthropological and psychological models of dissociation) the dialogue attempted here attempts to further join up such areas of research and critical thinking in a way not previously attempted. As such our models are of course provisional, but hopefully throw up important further avenues of exploration, for ethnography, psychology, cultural neuroscience and intervention (at both individual, group and population levels).

Ultimately we would hope the kind of scientifically informed, culturally sensitive formulation advanced here might assist in the design and implementation of culturally sensitive interventions for the distress endured by individuals with brief recurrent psychosis, which of course might include a facilitated return to traditional models of healing (cf. Gone 2013), in which the cultural realities discussed are already implicit and embedded.

1.2 Methodology

The research was split over two sites: Becora, a *Suco* (suburb) of the capital, Dili; and Hera a semi-rural farming, community 30 km from Dili. Both sites had been profoundly affected by the atrocities of 1999, and Becora in particular, a densely housed suburb of Dili, had been razed to the ground.

We have described our methodology more fully elsewhere (Silove et al. 2008) and will emphasize here aspects most relevant to the current discussion. Two case-finding methods were employed, going from household to household, across an entire community, and using census data to ensure coverage. The first used standardised and widely applied psychological screening tools in cross-cultural settings, the *Kessler Psychological Distress Scale* (K10; Patel et al. 2008; Sulaiman-Hill and Thompson 2010) and the *Harvard Trauma Questionnaire* (HTQ; Mollica et al. 1992; Renner et al. 2006), comparable with the previous study done in the wake of the 1999 atrocities (Modvig et al. 2000), which between them cover a range of experienced distress but with a strong emphasis on traumatic experiences and their psychological consequences.

The second case finding method utilised a novel community approach to case identification that invoked local idioms of madness, previously established through extensive community liaison, questionnaires and focus groups (Graves 2003) and then piloted again for content validity, as a means to find potential cases of serious mental distress and illness, in addition to helping us understand what types of problem the community perceives to fall within this category (Silove et al. 2008). The local Tetum idioms used were: (1) *bulak*—a generic but somewhat pejorative term for madness; (2) *pontu*—another generic idiom but which appeared to emphasize the observation of nonsensical speech; (3) *hanoin barak*—literally translated as "thinking too much", and therefore tempting to equate with PTSD, but colloquially sometimes used as a less pejorative version of *bulak*; (4) *bilan*—implying an "empty mind" and colloquially used to denote people with an apparent intellectual disability; (5) *fulan lotuk*—the dark moon or late waning/early waxing crescent moon (literally "slim moon"), denoting both idiom and explanatory model of perceived causality. Respondents were also given the opportunity to provide other terms to identify community or family members perceived to have mental health problems.

Sub-samples of individuals from both groups were then subject to a more vigorous clinical diagnostic interview using the Structured Clinical Interview for DSM-IV-TR (SCID) (First et al. 2002), administered by two British trained doctors with postgraduate training in psychiatry, and undergraduate degrees in medical anthropology, and a third Australian trained doctor with postgraduate experience in psychiatry, directly supervised by the former. Impairment and disability ratings were also made according to the SCIDs Global Assessment of Function (GAF) and the World Health Organization Short Disability Assessment Schedule[6] (WHO DAS-S—Janca et al. 1996). Burden of disease assessments were also initially attempted utilising the Zarit Burden interview schedule (Lim et al. 1996; Magana et al. 2007; Zarit et al. 1980) although were not persisted with for reasons later discussed (see Sect. 5.2.1).

The qualitative component utilised a modified version of the Short Explanatory Model Interview (SEMI—Lloyd et al. 1998), a short semi-structured interview, based on Kleinman's (1978) concept of explanatory models that attempts to elicit the name and nature of the identified problem, alongside perceived causes and consequences covering multiple domains of influence—from the physical, through the socio-economic, to the supernatural. Help seeking behaviour is also enquired about, alongside expectations of outcome. We reframed initial questions from the original SEMI to fit a research, rather than clinical context, and illness vignettes were not used. The SEMI uses open-ended questions, followed by closed probes, to explore possible attributions and consequences not mentioned spontaneously, although spontaneous descriptions were accorded more significance in our analysis (cf. Jadhav et al. 2001). In our study attribution probes were derived from the earlier

[6]For inter-episodic patterns of distress we based this on the worst period of functioning which while an important marker of severity would have significantly inflated the perception of overall impairment, particularly for sufferers of very brief episodes.

qualitative study (Graves 2003) and pilot, and initial interviews. The closed probes used for illness attribution in our study were: (1) physical causes; (2) breaking traditions or violating the sacred (Tetum: *lulik*); (3) past trauma; (4) social problems; (5) the dark/crescent moon (Tetum: *fulan lotuk*); (6) heredity; (7) accident; (8) due to spirits (Tetum: *rai nain* or *bai nain*—earth or water spirits, literally "lords of the land/water"). Probes in relation to consequences were: (1) social difficulties; (2) home difficulties; (3) work difficulties; (4) married life/marriage prospects.

Where possible however, and before any closed questioning, sufficient time was afforded for elicitation and engagement with open ended *illness narratives* (cf. Kleinman 1988) and indeed our richest qualitative data came from the more open-ended, fluid conversations, which preceded clinical assessment (see Sect. 1.7.1).

1.3 Ethnographic Context

Our engagement with the local community and qualitative research process, with indigenous colleagues acting as culture-brokers, provided us with important insights into local customs and belief. Although this process fell well short of the full ethnographic immersion we were able to supplement our cultural knowledge with the insights from historical and contemporary ethnography. The use of such material presented its own dilemmas since historically the longstanding inhabitants of Timor are made up of a great diversity of ethnolinguistic groups, particularly on the East of the island, where it is estimated at least fifteen distinct languages are spoken by different groups (see Fig. 1.1; Fox 1996; Taylor-Leech 2009) and our own research reflects this diversity. Within the narrower psychotic cohort forming our current focus (see Sect. 1.4.2—Table 1.1) a third was made up of primary Tetum speaking groups,[7] and all but one (with two unknowns) were primary speakers of Austronesian derived languages (the exception was one Fataluku speaker which belongs to the "Trans New Guinea Phylum of languages" (McWilliam 2007, 355) who came from a household were Tetum was also spoken). This is significant since research has demonstrated that Austronesian-based language speakers share some common cultural origins and influences, impacting at the level of local belief and practice (Bellwood, Fox, and Tryon 1995), and indeed even Fataluku speakers—on account of a long history of Austronesian cultural engagement and fusion, have been caricatured "Austronesians in disguise" (McWilliam 2007, 355).

Additionally while the cultural resistance and resilience of East Timorese peoples in the face of five hundred years of Portuguese contact and later Indonesian

[7]We did not distinguish in our study between the more widely spoken *Tetum-Praça* (also known as *Tetum-Dili* or "market Tetum"), *Tetum-Terik* (also known as *Classical Tetum*) and Tetum-*Belu* (spoken on each side of the East–West border); although given overall usage, and our proximity to the capital Dili, it is likely that where Tetum was identified as the language spoken at home, it more often referred to the *Tetum-Praça* (Kingsbury 2010; Taylor-Leech 2008).

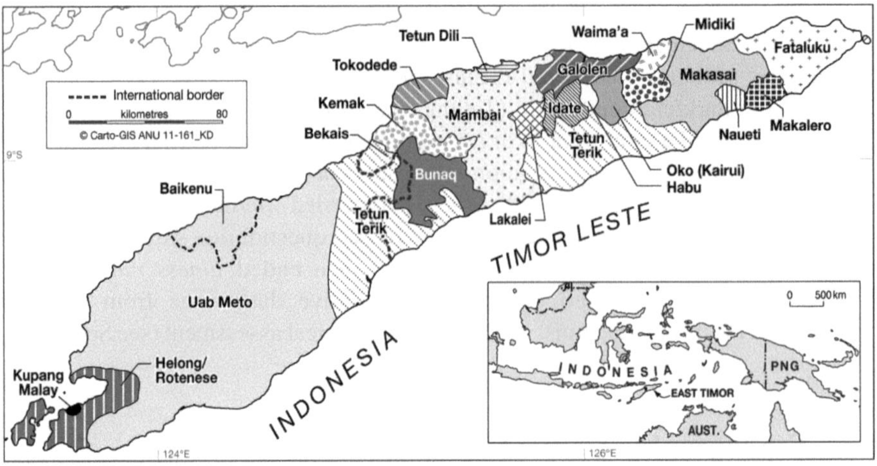

Fig. 1.1 Ethnolinguistic map. The ethnolinguistic map used with permission from the Australian National University uses Dutch spelling of local dialects in contrast to the Portuguese used throughout this work. TheAustralianNationalUniversity,CAPCartoGIS

occupation is well established (Carey 1999; Gunn 2001), widespread displacement and intermixing of different cultural groups during Indonesian times, accompanied by a growing fervent Nationalism and the adoption of Tetum as a language of resistance and later as an official lingua franca, has further reinforced links between different ethnolinguistic groups[8] (Taylor-Leech 2008). The growing influence of the Catholic church is similarly likely to have had some cultural ramifications, although Fox (1996) argues that even before the Catholicism became widely adopted during the Indonesian period as a symbol and bastion of resistance (see Sect. 2.3.1). Catholic emissaries had long been tolerated as their teachings appeared broadly compatible with existing Tetum understandings of gendered power and divinity, into which they were assimilated.

We nonetheless recognise the limitations of such forces of cultural convergence. Not least, as Traube (2011) reminds us, is the distinction between views of Nationalism as bestowed and proclaimed from *above*, and as understood and contested from *below*. In addition, at times of economic scarcity, civil conflict is often played out along, and tends to reinforce ethnolinguistic lines, as was the case in Timor-Leste in 2006 (Durand 2009; see Sect. 4.1.1).

Nonetheless overall, we have felt justified on drawing upon relevant ethnographic material pertaining to Timor-Leste to help us further illuminate the cultural backdrop, although the material available was further limited by the large

[8]In terms of National identity it is significant that the new post-Independence government officially decreed that "there is to be a distancing from Indonesian-influenced [Tetum- Praça] idiom in favour of Tetum- Terik, which has fewer modern Indonesian loanwords" (Taylor-Leech 2008, 161; see Footnote 7 above) in an attempt to offset forces of acculturation (see also Sect. 4.2.3).

"ethnographic gap" between 1975 and 1999 on account of barriers to social-science research during Indonesian rule[9] (McWilliam and Traube 2011a, 9). There is also little specific work in psychiatric anthropology in Timor-Leste, although Sakti's (2013) work on non-psychotic illness is an important exception. Beyond this, we have made efforts, in discussion with colleagues and key local consultants, to confirm the continued relevance of ethnographic work, and not to extend our arguments beyond that which we can find justification for. Given that our analysis draws on broader Timorese and Austronesian themes, alongside our desire to further protect the personal identities of individuals described in our case-histories, we have not identified the narrower ethnolinguistic identities of these individuals (see Ethics section below).

Ethics

The Human Research Ethics Committee of The University of New South Wales and the Timor-Leste Ministry of Health approved the study, along with the local community leaders of each area. Verbal consent was obtained from participants on account of low literacy levels in much of the population in the study. While always a difficult balance between confidentiality and provision of necessary context, as stated in the front matter, in order to preserve the anonymity of persons described in case material, names, specific location, *narrow* ethnolinguistic grouping, and other sensitive identifying features have been changed or withheld. We believe we have achieved this with minimal compromise to more essential material necessary for our analysis. In addition there seemed an evident possibility in relation to a couple of case histories that intra-familial abuse might have occurred. Due to the sensitivity of this subject in Timor-Leste we have not directly drawn attention to this in the commentary to these cases and have left it to the reader to draw their own conclusions.

An advocacy-based model of research was also deployed in that, where possible, attempts were made to secure help for anyone found to be suffering from significant emotional or mental health difficulties, within the limits imposed by the existing service and health infrastructure. In practice this usually meant referral to government health services or NGOs.

[9]The majority of detailed ethnographic work had been done in Timor-Leste prior to the Indonesian occupation of 1975 (e.g. Forman 1977; Hicks 2004; Traube 1986) although an array of shorter works of usually of circumscribed focus are now starting to appear based on post-Independence research (e.g. Bovensiepen 2009; McWilliam and Traube 2011b [edited vol.]; Traube 2007). Our leaning on, and comparison of, two major two major pre-Indonesian ethnographies relating to Austronesian speaking peoples, the Tetum (Hicks 2004) and the Mambai (Traube 1986), confirmed many common themes in belief and practice, although we acknowledge significant differences too.

1.4 Results

1.4.1 Overview

The *quantitative* results of this study have been presented more fully elsewhere (Silove et al. 2008). In summary we identified 1544 adults living in 548 dwellings. We achieved 100 % coverage of households for the community-identified arm of the study and an 82.4 % population response rate for the screening arm.

124 participants (10 %) of the screened population scored above threshold on one or both screening measures, 44 % of whom were subject to more in depth qualitative and diagnostic interviews as described. 30 participants were also identified via the community-identified route, only 6 of whom overlapped with the screen-positive cohort. Of this group, full histories were taken in relation to 23 of the subjects with the remainder in the main, being too unwell to participate and/or untraceable. All had obvious mental health difficulties, although experienced and articulated through local cultural idioms, and in all but 2 of this group, it was possible to formulate a DSM-IV diagnosis to sit alongside local understandings (Silove et al. 2008).

Combining both case-finding methods, we identified a point prevalence of those meeting DSM-IV criteria for PTSD of 1.47 % (n = 8), for depression of 1.64 % (n = 10), and for alcohol abuse or dependence of 0.62 % (n = 5). We also identified a point prevalence of *broadly defined psychosis* of 1.35 % (n = 16)—although only 0.34 % (n = 4) of this group was constituted by those meeting diagnostic criteria for schizophrenia, and 0.17 % (n = 2) by those meeting criteria for bipolar disorder—the rest, 0.84 % (n = 10) falling into the broader category of *psychotic disorder not otherwise specified* (*PDNOS*; see Sect. 1.5). Indeed of the 2 cases described as having bipolar disorder, one was atypical and classified as *bipolar disorder not otherwise specified* (*BPNOS*; see discussion in Sect. 1.5, Footnote 14).

Significantly all cases of psychosis were identified through the community-identified arm of the study and all cases of PTSD and depression were identified through the screening arm. While roughly a third of the community-identified psychosis would also have been picked up by the screening arm, none of those who met criteria for PTSD, and only 2 individuals with a primary depression, were picked up through the community-identified arm,[10] one of whom had mood-congruent psychotic features (see discussion in Sect. 1.6 incl. Footnote 23).

While the total population size of the survey region precludes overly confident estimates of low prevalence presentations (i.e. psychoses—see Sect. 1.6, incl. Footnote 17) a number of broad conclusions seem warranted from the survey consistent with wider cross-cultural research (Sect. 5.2):

[10]Apparent minor inconsistencies between actual case numbers and prevalence figures, between diagnostic groups, are attributable to denominator differences depending on the principle case-finding method.

- *Relatively* high rates of brief psychosis/psychotic disorder NOS—0.84 %
- *Comparatively* low rates of chronic psychosis (schizophrenia or bipolar)—0.51 %
- *Relatively* low rates of PTSD—1.47 %

1.4.2 Brief-Remitting-Relapsing Psychotic Phenomena

It was from the community case finding method and follow-up interviews, that the relatively frequent phenomena forming the focus of this paper were recorded: relatively *brief but severe and recurrent* episodes of acute mental and behavioural disturbance suggestive of psychosis (n = 10). Triggers for such episodes or exacerbations, included the more culturally familiar (to us) family and social stressors (clearly reported in 6/10), but also more culturally novel *lulik* triggers such as the time of the new/crescent moon (Tetum: *fulan lotuk*) which was reported as a notable and often recurrent trigger to psychotic phenomena in 7/10 in this group (see Sect. 2.3.4—Table 2.1). A further unanticipated feature, described by half the cohort, was disavowal or amnesia, on the part of the protagonist, of any recollection of the disturbed behaviour.

Table 1.1 Frequency of demographic factors and case finding methods

Demographic factor	Acute-remitting (n = 10)	Acute-on-chronic (n = 4)
Suco		
• Becora (urban)	4	2
• Hera (rural)	6	2
Age		
• 20–29	3	
• 30–39	1	1
• 40–59	5	
• >60	1	3
Sex		
• M	5	2
• F	5	2
Education		
• None/informal	4	4
• Primary	2	
• Secondary	2	
• Higher	2	
Occupation		
• None/domestic duties	3	1
• Subsistence farming	4	
• Market/street seller		3
• Labourer	1	
• Student	1	
• Healer	1	

(continued)

Table 1.1 (continued)

Demographic factor	Acute-remitting (n = 10)	Acute-on-chronic (n = 4)
Relationship status		
• Single	2	
• Married	7	1
• Widowed	1	2
• Divorced		1
Languages spoken at home		
• Tetum	4	1
• Mambai (+Tetum)	2	1
• Lolein (+Tetum)	2	
• Fataluku (+Tetum)	1	0
• Naueti (+Tetum)	1	2
• Unknown primary language		
Community identified terms		
• Bulak	5	3
• Pontu	1	4
• Hanoinbarak	2	1
• Fulan Lotuk	3	2
• Bilan	0	
Screen positive		2 not screened
• HTQ	0	0
• K10	4	0

Table 1.2 Episode characteristics

Episode characteristic	Acute-remitting/10	Acute-on-chronic/4
Inter-episodic recovery		
• Able to work	9	3
• Able to help at home	1	1
Triggers		
• New/Crescent moon ☾	7	4
• Social stress	6	2
Frequency (average)		
• Daily or greater	2	1
• Weekly	1	1
• Weekly–monthly	2	2
• Monthly	3	
• >Monthly (>3 × per year)	2	
Onset		
• 1975–1980	1	
• 1980s	2	2
• 1990–1998	2	2
• 1999–2004	5	

(continued)

Table 1.2 (continued)

Episode characteristic	Acute-remitting/10	Acute-on-chronic/4
Duration (episodes)		
• Several hours	3	
• 1–2 days		1
• 3–5 days	4	1
• Variable (5 days—one month)	1	
• Uncertain (but less than 10 days)	2	2

Table 1.3 Symptom frequencies

Symptom	Acute-remitting-relapsing (n = 10)	Acute-on-chronic (n = 4)
Psychomotor agitation	10	3
Irritability	9	3
Disorganised speech	8	4
Hallucinations (any)	8	3
• Auditory	4	3
• Tactile	3 (+1 historical)	1
• Visual	1 (+1 historical)	0
Aggression	6	3
• Verbal (only)	4(2)	3(0)
• Destructive of property	5	1
• Interpersonal violence	3	3
Easily angered (inter-episodic)	5	3
Amnesia (post-episode)	5	1
↑somatic symptoms (acute)	5	1
Insomnia (acute)	5	0
Delusions (any)	4	4
• Persecutory	1	0
• Of reference	0	2
• Grandiose	1	1
• Other	2	1
Anxiety (acute)	4	0
Paranoid ideation	4	4
Disorganised behaviour	3	1
Pressured speech	3	0
>3 symptoms of mania	3	0
Confusion/perplexity	3	0
>3 symptoms of depression (inter-episodic)	3	0
Inappropriate affect	2	2
Hypersomnia (post-episode)	2	0

Brief-remitting-relapsing (BRR) psychotic (or psychotic-like) presentations (designated PDNOS; see Sect. 1.5) accounted for over half of all psychotic presentations, making up a quarter of all diagnoses. The frequency of various demographic characteristics, triggers and other episode characteristics are shown in Tables 1.1 and 1.2. In summary male and female prevalence were equal. While age was widely distributed the modal age range was 40–59. Urban and semi-rural inhabitants were roughly equally represented. There was a spread of educational levels and occupations, but the majority were uneducated and had no formal occupation. The majority were married, although 3 were widowers; there was only 1 divorcee. There majority were primary Tetum speakers, although all others could speak Tetum as an additional dialect. All cases were identified via the community-identified method and *Bulak* was the most common community identified term used to describe these states of mind and associated behaviours. 4 persons were also concurrently identified via psychological screening.

The descending frequency of various symptoms can be clearly seen in Table 1.3. Of particular note was the ubiquitous presence of agitation, although subjective anxiety was less commonly verbalised. Disorganised speech (Tetum: *koalia arbiru* or *koalia nar-naran deit*—talking randomly) was also extremely common. Hallucinations were common and apparent in different modalities. Verbal aggression and destruction of property were reported by half the sample, and half were "quick to anger" (Tetum: *hirus lalais)*, but actual interpersonal violence appeared less common. Acute insomnia was reported in half the sample and in 2 of these person's post-episode hypersomnia was described—both also associated with subsequent amnesia/disavowal of the mental state and behaviour in question. Paranoid or persecutory ideas were seen in half the sample. In a small number there were concurrent confusion/perplexity (3/10), subthreshold manic symptoms (3/10 —but see discussion in Sect. 1.5, Footnote 14) or inter-episodic symptoms of depression (3/10—crossing diagnostic threshold for 1 subject: see Sect. 4.1.2—Case BP6), but at a subthreshold level in the other 2 individuals).

A list of nominal SCID-generated DSM-IV diagnosis is provided in Table 1.4—the most common being PDNOS, with one case of BPNOS. One instance of PDNOS described below was associated with alcohol dependence, although not clearly causally related to this (as evidenced by a period of abstinence—see Case BP1 below). In 2 of the PDNOS cohort an organic cause could not be categorically

Table 1.4 Diagnosis

SCID generated DSM-IV diagnosis	Acute-remitting-relapsing (n = 10)	Acute-on-chronic (n = 4)
• None	1	
• Psychotic disorder NOS (type 1)	6	
• Bipolar disorder NOS	1	
• Schizophrenia		2
• Psychotic disorder NOS (type 5) or due to GMC	2	2

excluded and as such were designated PDNOS subtype 5. One of these persons, a man, suffered with concurrent alcohol dependence with intermittent psychotic-like bizarre symptoms (see Sect. 4.2.2—Case BP7); the other, a woman, described a history of equivocal head-injury contemporaneous with the onset of psychotic-like symptoms (see Sect. 2.3.4—Case BP5). One case did not meet criteria for a formal DSM-IV diagnosis (see Sect. 1.5.1 and 2.3.2–Case BP2). At least half of the cases had been ill for five years or more.

In terms of diagnosis, it was apparent that persons with very similar BRR presentations were found to cut across diagnostic groups. We have therefore included all subjects presenting with BRR *disordered speech and behaviour* (except where clearly *solely* attributable to alcohol misuse), regardless of diagnosis in our analysis, in our efforts to construct an overlapping psychosocial and cultural formulation around such behaviour.

Demographics (including frequency of cultural idioms), episode characteristics (duration, triggers, frequency etc.), symptom frequencies and SCID generated DSM-IV diagnoses, are tabulated in Tables 1.1, 1.2, 1.3 and 1.4.

Case BP1—A Brief-remitting-relapsing Psychotic Pattern in a 30 Year Old Man:
Adriano, a 30 year old single male, lived with relatives and was unemployed, although worked on the family farm making traditional alcohol when well. He was identified by the local community as "fulan lotuk." We were told by family members that during the new moon he became generally more irritable and restless, appeared to laugh and talk to himself, and had a propensity towards violence and destruction of property. These "sickness" episodes were reported as occurring two to three times a month, lasting for up to four days, including, invariably, at the time of the new moon, at which times his behaviour was reported as particularly disturbed. Outside of these times, his family were unanimous in their view that his behaviour was "completely normal" and he was able to work in the fields and contribute to household duties. There was little consensus within the family as to when the problem started but the most conservative estimate was in the previous five years. No one recalled an obvious precipitant of the problem. Like many Timorese, Adriano fled to the mountains during the 1999 tragedy before eventually ending up in his home town 100 km away. This was not accorded any significance however, and his family say that he did not witness or experience any significant trauma, and was not separated from them while away from home. On the HTQ trauma screening questionnaire previously distributed, Adriano had been recorded as saying that he had been witness to the murder of family and/or friends but he later denied this and his family reported that there was no truth in this.

During the more direct, structured, SCID-based interview Adriano and his family reflected that he often felt very sad, tearful and "empty inside." He did not appear to meet criteria for a depressive episode for although he sometimes experienced other associated symptoms, these were only fleeting, although at interview he appeared to show little variation in affect.

According to the family the first sign that a sickness episode was coming on was that Adriano would begin to talk to himself, as if interacting and responding, or laughing to himself for no apparent reason. His family reported that when unwell his speech would get very muddled ("koalia arbiru"—lit. random speech), which we clarified as meaning sentences may be unrelated to one another, or may make no sense at all. Responding to direct questioning, one family member agreed that he sometimes used made up words and the family agreed that he talked faster and a lot more than usual. During these periods Adriano had been noted to become physically very restless, being unable to sit still and often wandering around aimlessly, during both day and night. He reportedly slept a great deal less than normal, averaging three to four hours a night. Further focused questions however elicited no suggestion of grandiosity, distractibility, risk-taking or other symptoms suggestive of mania.

When in this state he was described however as extremely irritable ("hirus lalais"—lit. quick to anger) and if challenged or interrupted, there was concern that he might become aggressive and violent. He spontaneously challenged people who were in his vicinity and had frequently gotten into fights. On such occasions, he reportedly wouldn't hesitate to grab a sharp implement to use as a weapon, and his aunt believed it was a miracle no one had so far has been hurt. He could also become very destructive of property and had, in recent times before our visit, reportedly attempted to burn down his brother's house. His targets have also included seemingly purposeless objects or innocent animals. On one occasion he bit his teeth into a tree. On others he has killed random animals and tore the foetus out of a pregnant sow without obvious motive. His family say they have never tried to physically restrain him and that they have realized a "softly-softly" approach— giving into his demands and being very patient around him—is the only way to manage his aggression. They say the police have not been involved directly in any incidents but rather on many occasions Adriano himself has called the police alleging there to be unrest in the area unapparent to others. No further evidence of other unusual beliefs was uncovered. When the sickness episodes passed he would reportedly sleep heavily for several days and on waking he would usually deny full recollection of the said events.

We attempted to interview Adriano himself on two occasions. On the first occasion rapport was hard to establish and he made mainly single word replies to most questions, describing his problem repetitively, as "something that comes on inside making him tense" which he agreed, on clarification, was sometimes associated with sweating and palpitations. On the second occasion he was even harder to engage (his family felt he might be becoming unwell) and he appeared perplexed by our presence. We encountered Adriano unintentionally on a further occasion, during an interview with a different subject in the same neighbourhood, during which Adriano stumbled onto the veranda appearing agitated and demanding medicine from us, before being shepherded away by a neighbour. During our conversations in the main Adriano denied disturbed behaviour or psychotic experiences, although acknowledged occasional voice-hearing experiences. These included hearing a voice call out his name. We were unable to discover much more except that he seemed clear that the voices do not comment on his actions or talk to each other.

During further direct questioning his family said they thought he was sometimes feverish after such episodes, although never at other times and the picture was complicated by probable alcohol dependence. Although difficult to elicit he gave a history of physical dependence symptoms—autonomic hyperactivity, tremor, insomnia, gastrointestinal symptoms, agitation, anxiety and visual hallucinations on withdrawal, and tolerance—he acknowledged he knowingly drank to avoid getting sick. He said he also found it hard to stop despite acknowledging that it appeared to aggravate his mental condition. He further complained of "burning pains" inside his stomach, which were not limited to times when he was mentally unwell. He reported he consumed about one litre of traditional alcohol (palm wine) a day until, in recent times before our visit, he had apparently managed to cut down because of more frequent sickness episodes. There was no clear relationship evident however, between his acute sickness episodes, and cycles of intoxication or withdrawal. On our advice, with the help of Timor-Leste's first community detox, and with subsequent family enforcement he apparently managed to stop drinking altogether—although the sickness episodes reportedly continued until he was placed on a low dose of antipsychotic medication by the local mental health workers.

We will return to a commentary on this case (see Sects. 3.1.1, 3.1.3, 4.2.2 and 4.23) alongside others throughout this book.

1.4.3 Acute-on-Chronic Psychotic Exacerbation

A further 4 cases were described in which pre-existing chronic psychotic symptoms and behaviour, was exacerbated at the time of the *fulan lotuk*. In 2 out of these 4 cases exacerbation was also associated with family and social stress. The small number makes any demographic or clinical comparison unreliable, although they tended to be older, widowed and more likely to be working outside the home (most often engaged in subsistence street or market selling). Other demographic variables were not notably different (see Table 1.1).

In these cases of acute-on-chronic (AOC) psychotic exacerbation, symptom profiles were not radically different from the BRR group, although voice hearing was the dominant hallucinatory modality. There was less evidence of subjective anxiety or mood disturbance (although agitation and irritability remained common) and episodes of interpersonal violence were more common (see Table 1.3). 2 subjects in this group met DSM-IV criteria for schizophrenia (Cases CP1 and CP3). A third was further classified as PDNOS (subtype 5) on account of a history of chronic recurrent fever (Case CP2) that rendered us "unable to determine whether [the psychosis] was primary, [or] due to a general medical condition" (First et al. 2002, 96). A forth appeared to have dementia (with psychotic features) secondary to head injury (Case CP4) although this was not diagnosable via the SCID algorithm —the closest classification being *psychotic disorder due to a general medical condition*—and although included here (see Table 2.1), she was excluded from epidemiological analysis previously presented (Silove et al. 2008). However as with the BRR group, culturally influenced fluctuations in symptomatology, cut across diagnostic groups, but serve to illustrate the overlapping psychosocial and cultural formulation around such exacerbations.

We also note that there were 5 other subjects—2 meeting criteria for schizophrenia; 1 for bipolar I disorder; 1 for depression with secondary mood-congruent psychotic features; and 1 for PDNOS (again subtype 5)—all with chronic symptoms and impairment but not included in the AOC cohorts. This was on account of an absence, or else inadequate information to determine the presence, of culturally patterned fluctuations.[11]

Primarily for illustrative purposes we include a case-example from the AOC cohort below about which we will also offer brief further commentary in the final chapter (see Sect. 5.2.1). Assessment of this person required careful cultural calibration since the convoluted temporal narrative (jumping back and forwards in time in a manner sometimes difficult to follow) interspersed with elements of what from a literary Western perspective might be designated as *magical realism* were also apparent in the mythological narratives elicited by Traube (2007; see Sect. 4.1.1) in her ethnographic fieldwork with Mambai-speakers in the mountainous district of Aileu. Nonetheless his speech and behaviour were identified by the community as idiosyncratic, he was subject to anomalous experiences, and his social and wider functioning was compromised to at least some degree suggesting his presentation did not fall into accepted cultural norms.

Case CP1: Acute-on-chronic Psychotic Exacerbation in a 60 Year Man
Christiano appeared to be in his 60s and was described by his co-resident daughters as "a little 'bulak'" and "a little 'pontu.'" They reported that he "talks a lot of nonsense" and that he was worse during the 'fulan lotuk'. He was previously married but, uniquely for the cohort under discussion here, divorced in 1989 as apparently his wife didn't accept his behaviour suggesting he may have had mental

[11]However both the individual with the bipolar presentation, and the individual with chronic and severe "psychotic depression" had notable histories of trauma and loss and described *lulik* factors around the time of onset, consistent with our hypothesis (see Sect. 2.3). The individual with the bipolar-presentation had long been on depot anti-psychotic medication, potentially minimising any fluctuation. The individual with psychotic-depression, described continuous symptoms, particular when alone or unoccupied, and while not describing culturally-influenced exacerbations the rapid *sealing-over* of her symptoms and distress when in company (including in our interview with her) and observed rapid *unsealing* of these when left alone appeared a striking example of the more general dissociative model developed here. In another individual, we were able to elicit sufficient information to indicate the criteria for schizophrenia were met, but the person was too aggressive towards us to enable either interview of him or his family in further detail about patterns of fluctuation—although the observation that his hostility and feelings of persecution were particularly directed at foreigners was no doubt of symbolic significance—see also Sect. 4.2.3). The other individual meeting criteria for schizophrenia had become deaf during childhood secondary to a febrile illness and also appeared to have a global intellectual disability, likely due to the same childhood illness. The forth individual, had a history of psychotic symptoms meeting criteria for schizophrenia although these reportedly began within days after being beaten unconscious by Indonesian soldiers and therefore a significant organic cause could not be excluded (PDNOS type 5).

health difficulties for some time. His daughters report that their earliest memories of him were that he was "bulak" although until 1984 he is understood to have had a responsible job in charge of workmen, and before that he worked as a cook.

On interview Christiano was fixated on events that occurred during 1966 and narrated his story in a very chaotic manner, shifting frames of reference, and jumping to parts of story or material that appeared to both family and interviewer/interpreter as tangential. Within this however it was possible to discern the bones of a story about a dispute in which he was accused of making a promise to marry a housekeeper, resulting in a row between her boss and his, the involvement of the police, and his eventual dismissal after an argument with his boss's wife. His daughter thought that some of these events may have occurred but that he had become fixated on them and that he acted as though people may still be talking and angry about him now.

He had some unusual beliefs but which appear within the limits of cultural acceptability, such as memories of seeing a "rai nain" (Tetum meaning land-spirit; literally "land lord") in the form of a snake while with a boy called Maubere—which he thought may have portended the later emergence of the "Maubere political party" but the "rai nain" took his soul.[12]

Following the direct and structured questioning of the SCID however, took us outside of this cultural frame. He was described as often being seen to talk to himself when alone and curse things that others cannot see (or sometimes real animals), or talk with the radio. He admitted to fairly frequent voice-hearing experiences, sometimes of men, sometimes of women, that may say to him things like "why are you walking", or "don't climb that tree" although generally he finds their advice helpful and the voices are never derogatory. No third person hallucinations or running commentary were apparent. He reported that the agents of the voices however do occasionally touch him—for example on the ribs—which he believes is on account of them trying to surprise him. When he turns round there is no one there. He said he had never seen them except in his dreams.

His daughters reported that he sometimes wanders around aimless, but this is confined to his home and apparently to daytime hours. Functionally he manages to a degree, and laughed when he said that he is "more than happy" because he is

[12]His daughter accepts he saw a *rai nain* but not that it tool his soul. It was not clear whether this was on account of *subtle* violations of cultural understandings of *rai nain* conduct (although we have read of similar accounts of *rai nain* behaviour in Hicks' (2004) ethnography) illness denial, or erosion of traditionally held beliefs in the younger generation (see Sect. 4.2.3). The "Maubere political party" may have referred to the National Council of Maubere Resistance, a chain in a series of political-paramilitary umbrella organisations that evolved into the National Council of Timorese Resistance, and ultimately negotiated terms for an Independence referendum (Niner 2001). As Traube (2007, 9) notes Maubere was originally a "common Mambai masculine name that was used during the Portuguese colonial period as a demeaning term of address for indigenous men" but which became appropriated and re-imagined by the ultimately victorious Fretlin political party as a potent symbol of and for "the people." As such it may have important significance for a psychotic individual (see also Sect. 4.1.1) struggling with rejection by both his wife and employer, although disentangling cause from effect, is of course now impossible.

"working hard" (selling betel nuts) rather than "riding in a car or an airplane". During this SCID-based questioning around his mood he noted however that he "feels worthless as an old man who has lost his power and energy" but he did not meet DSM criteria for a mood disorder, past or present. Significantly his daughter asserted that there are no obvious problems with his memory and on an impromptu and modified Mini Mental State Examination (MMSE) there were no obvious deficits.[13]

Case Numbering
Case histories have been numbered with the prefix BP- (brief-psychosis) where drawn from the *BRR* psychotic-cohort and CP- (chronic psychosis) where drawn from the *AOC* psychotic-exacerbation cohort. Occasionally we have presented case material from beyond the wider non-psychotic cohort to further illustrate particular points but this should be clear in the text and we have not further numbered these cases.

1.5 Classification

Symptom profiles, particularly for the BRR group tended to cut across traditional diagnostic groups, with aspects of both psychotic and affective disturbance commonly occurring together, the course or duration of which, however, was insufficient to justify a major conventional DSM-IV-TR (or indeed ICD-10 equivalent) psychiatric diagnosis of bipolar I disorder,[14] schizoaffective disorder or schizophrenia.

In terms of duration many of the brief-remitting presentations might more obviously have been classified, according to the SCID, as *brief psychotic disorders* (BPD; requiring complete resolution with four weeks), or if we had used ICD-10, as *acute and transient psychotic disorders* (ATPD; require resolution with 3 months). Additional features of BPD, not directly asked about by the SCID, but mentioned in the body of the text in DSM-IV-TR include "emotional turmoil", and "rapid shifts

[13]We did not have readily available access to cross-culturally validated screening tests of cognitive impairment so limited ourselves to impromptu questions of orientation, registration, attention, recall and language, derived from the MMSE in dialogue with an *interpreter-cum-culture-broker* to adjust for perceived cultural norms for an elderly, but in this instance, well-educated man. We also note the existence of studies supporting the modified use of the MMSE in similar contexts, including in an elderly and illiterate, rural, Indian population (Ganguli et al. 1995).

[14]The presence of paranoid ideation, grandiosity, delusions of reference and even disorganised speech and behaviour, alongside affective symptoms could be conceptualised as being compatible with a manic episode, and one subject (see Sect. 2.3.4—Case BP4) presenting with such symptoms could have had an episode classified in this way if utilising "irritability" as an entry criterion (A symptom) and counting "psychomotor agitation" as a secondary (B) symptom. Algorithmically however, such diagnostic alchemy feels less in keeping with conventional diagnostic understandings—a critique similar to that made against comparable and controversial diagnostic criterion modifications for so called "early onset bipolar disorder" in pre-pubertal children (Carlson 2005). To further complicate matters this person's further two episodes were of much shorter duration (4 days) but too disturbed (with psychotic symptoms) and impairing to be classified as hypomanic, suggesting at best, a poly-syndromal course within this system of classification (cf. Marneros and Pillmann 2004).

from one intense affect to another" (American Psychiatric Association (APA) 2000, 330). This might have been useful to directly enquire about and appeared consistent with our observations regarding a concurrent affective dimension to many of the BRR psychotic-like presentations described, but partly due to its rapid evolution, this was difficult to quantify.

Other symptoms, such as confusion (or perplexity), seen in the BRR group (3/9), are also acknowledged in the text of DSM-IV-TR, although are not invariable features of BPD. These features, overlap with that described for ATPD in ICD-10 (World Health Organisation (WHO) 1992), in particular the *acute polymorphic* subtypes which recognise the frequent co-manifestations of irritability and anxiety described in this cohort (in 9/10 and 4/10 respectively). However, polymorphism is also defined by rapid evolution in the intensity, content and modality of hallucinations or delusions, and for most of the BRR cohort, we did not have sufficient access to their internal worlds to confirm the nature of perceptual disturbance or unusual beliefs, instead often relying on observations and inferences made of their behaviour, in particular grossly disorganized speech or behaviour, but often including obvious responses to hallucinations. Because of these diagnostic-uncertainties the best-fit category from ICD-10 would have been the more generic "other ATPD" although the overarching ATPD-category as whole usefully allows for the narrower specification of an "abrupt onset" (within 48 h), since there is some evidence that "the more abrupt the onset, the better the outcome" (WHO 1992, Sect. F23). This additional descriptor of "abrupt onset" would in fact have applied to the entire BRR cohort in our study. In favour of DSM-IV (and also the more recent DSM-5—(APA 2013)) classification however is the due recognition of "disorganized speech (e.g., frequent derailment or incoherence)" and "grossly disorganized behavior" as standalone, entry symptoms, for a diagnosis of a BPD. *Indeed grossly disorganised speech and behaviour appeared prototypical—indeed idiomatic—of psychotic-states in Timor-Leste.*

Beyond their acute presentation, three of BRR cohort appeared to struggle with inter-episodic symptoms of depression, and one of these crossed the SCID's diagnostic threshold for *major depressive disorder* (see Sect. 4.1.2—Case BP6). This might suggest a formulation of a primary mood disorder with secondary psychotic symptoms ("psychotic depression") except there appeared no simple linear relationship between mood and episodic psychotic symptoms and onset of psychotic symptoms appeared more strongly associated with the culturally specific trigger of the *fulan lotuk* rather than mood severity. Additionally, and although not essential for a primary mood-related diagnosis, symptoms of disorganised speech and behaviour cannot obviously be conceptualised as mood congruent (unless perhaps taken to be an expression of nihilism, or perhaps from within a psychodynamic framework—see Sect. 3.2). More broadly, however, we will go onto argue that depressed or dysphoric mood can be better conceptualised as an additional risk factor for such brief-psychotic states within the formulation developed (see Sect. 5.3 incl. Fig. 5.1).

In partial recognition of the continuity of contemporary classification with earlier, Scandinavian influenced concepts, of *reactive* or *psychogenic* psychosis, DSM-IV/5 and ICD-10 all allow for an additional coding to enable suspected causal linkage with *culturally salient traumatic life-events* to be acknowledged, although difficulties in quantifying the impact of such events, alongside the avowedly theoretical nature of DSM-IV/5 in particular, have meant research in this area has been lacking, and depending on criteria of disorder and trauma used, findings have been highly variable (Singh 2011). Such coarse "everyman" definitions of "stress" are also not able to capture the kind of interactive, personal and cultural symbolic aspects of trauma advanced here, which do not fit with DSM-IV's concept of "events that, singly or together, would be markedly stressful to almost anyone in similar circumstances in the person's culture" (APA 2000, 330); definitions in DSM-5 and ICD-10 are comparable.

However in relation to our findings, a principle problem in all of the diagnostic criteria so far described is that the defining feature of the BRR group, namely *period recurrence* is not described, and while a benign relapsing course is a recognized trajectory of a subgroup of such cases within the wider research literature, intervals between such relapses are generally much longer (often discussed in years), particularly in developing country settings where such presentations are characterised by higher diagnostic stability and lower rates of relapse, vis-à-vis developed country settings (Castagnini and Berrios 2011). The higher frequency, even cyclical (and lunar-modulated) pattern of recurrence described in Timor-Leste, clearly lies outside of previously formally characterised trajectories and suggests the influence of additional, culture-related, factors on presentation.

Similarly, the commonly reported feature of post-episode amnesia (5/10) in the BRR cohort is not a recognised feature of brief psychosis in these standard diagnostic texts, which instead would point principally towards dissociative or organic disturbance or disorder (including intoxication) to account for this. Of course, in the context of our own study, it is important to note that dissociative disturbance is itself often described, in both DSM-IV/5 and ICD-10, in the context of *culture-related presentations* or *secondary to trauma* (in the latter including as a dimension of PTSD). While not without critique, of the 25 culture-bound syndromes described within the glossary of DSM-IV-TR, nine are described as having a *definite or possible dissociative dimension* (further demonstrating dissociative cultural pathoplasticity), and four include descriptions of psychotic-like or highly disorganized behaviour, reminiscent of our own cohort. One of these, *amok*, shares features, including post-episode hypersomnia (Hatta 1996; Kon 1994), with two of the more disturbed members of the BRR cohort (see Sect. 1.4.2—Case BP1 and Sect. 2.3.4—Case BP4), although in our study, in contrast to *amok*, significant violence or self-injury was rarely described (see Sect. 4.2.2).

We should point out, in terms of own work, although in common with many other epidemiological studies in this area (cf. Marneros and Pillmann 2004), the occurrence of brief-psychotic phenomena was not anticipated and the subtleties and atypical aspects described above were not probed through the SCID. Our understanding therefore evolved as the study progressed and if anything such features may therefore have been underreported. The advantage of our naivety was however the minimisation of expectation and theory-driven observer bias, thereby increasing our confidence in our overall clinical findings.

1.5.1 Culture of Diagnosis

While *DSM-IV/5* and the *ICD-10 Classification of Mental and Behavioural Disorders* is asserted to be atheoretical, its approach has been convincingly deconstructed to reveal a dominant biological framing of mental illness (Cooper 2004; Mezzich et al. 1999), that is mirrored in mainstream research (Read et al. 2001) and that simultaneously rests on dominant Euro-American cultural assumptions regarding the self, agency and responsibility (Gaines 1992). To this end, much contemporary theorising in relation to brief-psychotic episodes have recapitulated dominant ideas of genetic-biological vulnerability (cf. Marneros and Pillmann 2004), with older theories of psychogenesis no longer in vogue (Castagnini 2010; Jauch and Carpenter 1988).

Current concepts of BPD or ATPD of course have a rich pedigree and lineage in various European, including colonial and early post-colonial, schools of psychiatric thought. Research has indicated however that attempts to unite these diverse historical and cross-national formulations into the broader categories developed in DSM-IV/5 and ICD-10, might result in loss of construct and predicative validity, compared to some of their more regional precursors (Pillmann et al. 2000, 2003; see Sect. 5.2.5, incl. Footnote 21).

Additionally multiple competing diagnostic formulations from within, and beyond, these formal classifications might readily be suggested. For example, one of the younger women in the BRR cohort (Table 2.1—BP9), classified in Table 1.4 via the SCID as PDNOS, might have been more appropriately classified under the ICD-10 classification of *trance and possession disorder* (or the comparable operationalised research-criteria for *dissociative trance disorder* suggested in DSM-IV-TR–appendix B[15]). In ICD-10 (WHO 1992, Sect. F44.3) this classification is applied on account of:

> temporary loss of both the sense of personal identity and full awareness of the surroundings; … as if taken over by another personality, spirit, deity, or "force."… There is often a limited but repeated set of movements, postures, and utterances.

We should note that DSM-IV/5 and ICD-10 generally exclude culturally sanctioned responses and practices from their diagnostic landscape—including for trance and possession, although this is more clearly expounded and explicit in DSM-IV/5. For this reason, one member of the BRR cohort (see Sect. 2.3.2—Case BP2), remains unclassified, since his hallucinatory experiences and beliefs appeared in keeping with normative cultural parameters. He has been included in our discussion and case histories however because he continues to display, non-psychotic, verbally confronting behaviour at the time of *fulan lotuk* although his hallucinatory

[15]Operationalised research criteria for the sub-classification of *possession trance* also further specifies "full or partial amnesia for the event." (APA 2000, 785). *Dissociative trance disorder* was ultimately not included in DSM-5 although the concept is acknowledged and subsumed in the broader category of *Other Specified Dissociative Disorder* (APA 2013, 307).

experiences have long since ceased. He remains illustrative of our wider thesis, which is intended to transcend specific diagnostic groups.

To further muddy the diagnostic waters, it is of interest that in their combined literature review and prospective study of brief psychotic presentations (the latter admittedly not in a comparable cultural context), Marneros and Pillman (2004) identify core symptoms of: (i) abrupt (not just acute) onset; (ii) rapidly evolving symptom morphology (polymorphism); (iii) rapidly changing, including frequent bipolarity, of mood states; and (iv) anxiety. Taken together these are quite suggestive of a dissociative aetiology and bear an uncanny resemblance to historical descriptions of so called "hysterical psychosis" (cf. Hollender and Hirsch 1964; van der Hart et al. 1993) which have also reportedly found cross-cultural expression (Langness 1967). We are further impressed by the concept of "dissociative psychosis" advanced by van der Hart and Wiztum (2008), which might have been applied to many in the BRR cohort, although their concept is predicated on a narrow concept of "structural dissociation" (see Chap. 2), which while relevant, has less scope for the incorporation of constituent cultural factors, than advocated here (see Chap. 4).

In conclusion, for reasons of epistemological doubt and atypicality of presentation we have opted to categorise the BRR phenomena observed, according to the SCID, predominantly as PDNOS, or, in one case BPNOS (see Sect. 2.3.4—case BP4). Both essentially imply a *null diagnosis* that in our view *rightly* implies mental and behavioural phenomena poorly captured by existing concepts, and opening up the way for debate about their qualities (consistent with our first epigraph). Where presentations represent acute exacerbations of pre-existing, chronic distress and disturbance, the conventional diagnosis according to the DSM-IV-TR SCID algorithm has been noted in Table 1.4, although this should not imply uncritical endorsement of their nosological or cross-cultural validity.

Our emphasis in this work is on the development of a psychosocial and cultural formulation that contributes to an understanding of the unique temporal patterning and symptom profiles that cuts across conventional diagnostic categories. In this respect, questions about the "right diagnosis" are less important than an understanding of forms and patterns of distress in the wider individual and sociocultural context.

1.6 Commentary

As we have seen PTSD accounted for only 20 % of all diagnosis and its point prevalence estimated by our study in 2004 was 1.47 %—a finding that appeared exceptional in view of the countries occupied history and contingent widespread human rights violations, culminating in the humanitarian tragedy of 1999.[16]

[16]Very high rates of traumatic events were endorsed by the study population, using the cross-culturally validated and locally modified HTQ (see Sect 1.2), in which the mean number of traumatic events endorsed by any one individual was 4.2 (SD 2.61), with only 4.2 % of the population reporting no experience of trauma (Silove et al. 2009).

Alongside this finding we documented a point prevalence of chronic-psychosis of 0.51 % (combining schizophrenia—0.34 % and bipolar—0.17 %). While for methodological reasons generating confident quantitative estimates for low prevalence disorders and making comparisons of prevalence rates with Western developed nations is difficult, the prevalence of PTSD, schizophrenia and bipolar disorder appear lower than corresponding estimates in high-income countries[17] (Kessler et al. 1997, 2005; Saha et al. 2005) and in particular, the high ratio of BRR to chronic psychotic presentations appears striking.

Although the relationship between trauma and psychotic-reactions has been historically contested, there is now abundant evidence of a causal link, with even mainstream biologically oriented journals now coming cautiously on board (Cutajar et al. 2010; Read and Bentall 2012; Shevlin et al. 2008). A key question is how should the *relatively* high rates of BRR psychosis recorded in Timor-Leste be understood alongside the observation of the comparatively low rates of both PTSD and chronic psychosis (schizophrenia and bipolar disorder) at the time of our study. In this regard we contend that both socially learnt cultural practices that "favor dissociation over other coping strategies"[18] (Kirmayer 2011, 466) alongside early

---

[17]Prevalence rates may be reported as a point-, period-, or lifetime range, with use of lifetime prevalence often preferred for methodological reasons (Kessler 2000). For PTSD the closest we can get to the point prevalence used in our study is a twelve-month period prevalence, which in the United States, for PTSD, is estimated at 3.5 % in adults (Kessler et al. 2005). While period prevalence will over-estimate the point prevalence for PTSD and a diagnosis of PTSD only requires a one month period of continuous symptoms, in reality the disorder is often more chronic and there is unlikely to be a large discrepancy between such measures of prevalence, that would account for the relatively low prevalence in Timor-Leste from our initial study in 2004. Differences between these prevalence-types are likely to be smaller for schizophrenia and bipolar disorder on account of their chronicity. A study in the United States using comparable DSM-III-R criteria documented the 12-month prevalence of bipolar disorder as 0.37 % (Kessler et al. 1997). A meta-analytic review of schizophrenia prevalence studies reported back a cross-national median point-prevalence of 0.46 % but noted significantly higher combined prevalence rates in developed country settings (Saha et al. 2005). Although low prevalence presentations such as psychosis are difficult to reliably quantify our community-identified method (see Sect. 1.2) within a close-knit, island bound community, reduces the chance of missed cases. If movement between regions occurred it would have been unlikely to have been in the direction of net loss from the region of our study around the capital, Dili. However the more intriguing finding is the ratio of BRR to chronic psychosis and how this might be understood (see Sect. 5.2)

[18]While it is widely acknowledged that cultural practices may influence forms and frequency of dissociation, proving this *empirically* is difficult. For example Zatzick et al. 1994) attempt to demonstrate variations in the frequency of trauma-linked dissociation across cultural groups may have been hampered by a number of methodological difficulties including: (1) the use of broad cultural groupings (African–American, Caucasian and Hispanic) that may have been internally heterogeneous or, in the other direction, convergence between groups on account of shared identity and experience as Vietnam veterans; (2) reliance on self-report measures of trauma, which in the context of PTSD and dissociation may be unreliable, and biased either towards high or low recall, depending on whether symptoms were intrusive or sealed-over at the time of interview. This complicates the authors' conclusions that the higher rates of dissociative experience in the African–American group were accounted for entirely by higher rates of trauma-exposure rather than other factors that might have included sociocultural influences.

(childhood) and later repeated exposure to severe trauma and loss (Lanius et al. 2010), in the presence of diminished protective factors (family, community and cultural; Hoshmand 2007), that include compromised early infant-caregiver attachments (see Sect. 3.2; Liotti 2006), have shaped individual responses to trauma in Timor-Leste in the direction of an increased likelihood of dissociative symptomatology, that might include possession states but in particular the BRR dissociative–psychotic idiom, identified in our study. Secondly, we will argue at length, that the social, culturally informed response to dissociative–psychosis, may delimit its progression to chronic psychosis (see Sect. 5.2).

Returning to the first point—is there an association between the tendency towards dissociative responses and the low rates of PTSD documented in the broader survey (Silove et al. 2008)? One possible answer could be that since dissociative states are understood to be *culturally pathoplastic* (Spiegel et al. 2011) and that such states may be shaped by sociocultural factors into patterns of distress or disorder not recognised by Western diagnostic criteria (a.k.a. the culture bound syndromes), a process of direct substitution of BRR dissociative-psychotic states is occurring in place of PTSD.[19] However given that the r*elatively* high point-prevalence of BRR psychotic-presentations (0.84 %—captured as PDNOS or BPNOS) is still too small to account for the low prevalence of PTSD by a process of direct substitution, this answer alone will not suffice.

Another possibility is that a *general dissociative coping style* in the population is simultaneously promoting an *array of parallel dissociative-responses* that may include non-pathological and potentially adaptive responses not recognised as clinically problematic, that may indeed have directly subtracted from potential PTSD prevalence. This position overlaps with important cultural critiques of the presumed universality of PTSD concept for non-Western populations since PTSD was originally described and conceptualised in Western populations, who are argued to have very different conceptions of both self and trauma than non-Western persons,[20] which in turns influences how symptoms are engendered, experienced, understood and responded to—arguably in the direction of greater resilience (Bracken 2001; Elsass 2001; but see discussion on networks of obligation below).

While adding depth to our understanding such perspectives do not preclude the possibility that persons will present with symptoms of PTSD, although they do have implications for how such symptoms might be understood and responded to. A follow-up study by members of our group in 2011, following a highly troubling period of internal violence lasting from 2006 to 2008 (see Sects. 1.3 and 4.1.1), and based on comparable methods to the present work, reported much higher rates of

---

[19]To contextualise this argument, within Western populations we also know that individual responses to trauma (excluding, for now, psychosis) can be myriad, ranging from considerable resilience to transient distress and resolution, to adjustment reactions, PTSD, dissociative disorders, depression, anxiety disorders and substance misuse (Renner et al. 2007).

[20]Western persons may privilege individual experience and memory over the collective, compared to populations less influenced by Western culture who may, in contrast, privilege the collective over the individual (Bracken 2001; but see Sect. 1.7.2, Footnote 32.

PTSD (approaching 17 %) than recorded in 2004. Of course both screening checklists and more in-depth clinical interviews may overestimate the significance of PTSD symptoms for the population, on account of their "demand characteristics" characterised by Kagee (2004) as the process by which *respondents may become unduly sensitised to the nature of the disorder being assessed in standardised questionnaires*—whether through an direct suggestion, an eagerness to please, an expectation or material help, or else the endorsement of symptoms that while present may not be held to be locally significant or personally salient (Bracken et al. 1995; Miller et al. 2006). As such this critique could be equally levelled (at least to some degree) at both our 2004 study, and the subsequent follow-up in 2011, although we were careful to push beyond superficial symptom-endorsement to obtain first-hand accounts of experience (see Sect. 1.2).

Therefore the effects of such demand-characteristics in our own groups work are likely to be more modest compared to an earlier study that relied on simple population screening measures (in the absence of more in depth structured-diagnostic interview[21]) although since the 2011 study aimed to re-interview the same adult population approached by our team in 2004, the higher rates of apparent PTSD in this context could potentially reflect *increased socialisation into the trauma model* (also influenced by the impact of other research besides our own, the establishment of the fledgling National mental health service grounded in Western models of mental ill-health, and a number of NGOs offering intervention for trauma-related difficulties and distress). Such effects however may go beyond simple demand-characteristics, but through "looping effects" alter the direction (and even psychobiology) of culturally constituted experience (see Sect. 1.7.2; cf. Hacking 1999).

While these arguments all have some explanatory utility, we do not need to position the model of dissociation, or dissociative-psychotic phenomena, in opposition to that of PTSD. It is quite possible that PTSD and dissociative-psychotic phenomena can co-exist alongside each other, either within the population (due to the differing influences of divergent constitutional, trauma-related, and sociocultural factors impacting upon different individuals) or within the same individual (either serially or concurrently alongside dissociative-psychotic symptomatology[22]). Growing understanding of dissociative-mechanisms is also leading to changing

---

[21]One such study by Modvig et al. (2000), conducted in the immediate wake of the 1999 humanitarian tragedy, estimated a much higher prevalence of PTSD (in the region of 35 %) than our own, but relied on simple screening questionnaires with clinical cut-offs, that unlike ours were not followed-up with in-depth clinical interviews. Since in our study only 21 % of those meeting screening cut-off criteria for PTSD were shown to meet clinical caseness after in-depth structured clinical interview (Silove et al. 2008), it seems certain that earlier studies would have significantly over-estimated PTSD prevalence (Steel et al. 2009).

[22]For example, one large-scale Australian study exploring the link between delusion-formation and trauma documented that delusion-formation may occur either in the presence of absence of PTSD symptoms, but showed "that PTSD complicating exposure to trauma increases the likelihood of endorsement of delusional experience compared with trauma exposure without PTSD" (Scott et al. 2007, 34). Another pathway to co-occurrence is the commonly recognised phenomena of so called "post-psychotic PTSD" although analysis and intervention in this context, as the Morrison et al. (2003)

understandings of PTSD and indeed for Ross (2006, 2008) the whole pantheon of psychiatric disorders might be more helpfully re-conceptualised through the lens of dissociation-psychology.

From this perspective, a further explanation for the patterns of traumatic injury observed in post-conflict Timor-Leste, is the possibility that PTSD may have been presenting through a now recognised *dissociative subtype* (American Psychiatric Association (APA) 2013; Lanius et al. 2010; see Sect. 2.2.1) that may be less detectable through conventional screening instruments used in our study, such as the HTQ. This is because by definition, the intrusions and emotional hyperarousal characterising conventional PTSD, is *walled off* from awareness, in its dissociative subtype. A reduction in emotional-salience might also be reinforced by the observed cultural tendency (at the time of our original study) not to medicalise the consequences of trauma and social suffering.[23] However such walling-off may only be partially effective and as such the much higher rates of PTSD documented in Timor-Leste in the later study in 2011 might be attributable to a failure of this mechanism, leading to a breaking-through of distressing memories and associated emotions, following recurrent trauma and the ongoing associated loss of confidence in personal security (see Sect. 2.2)—in addition to erosion of the overarching meanings and narrative coherence of the Independence struggle that previously bound experiences of trauma to a wider vision of necessity, justified means and expected recompense[24] (see Sect. 4.1.1).

In addition, as Sakti (2013) points out, following her recent ethnographic fieldwork in the isolated Western Austronesian-Baiqueno speaking enclave of Oecussi (see Sect. 1.3—Fig. 1.1: Ethnolinguistic map), the response to trauma and loss in Timor-Leste needs to be understood not simply in terms of individual emotional distress and adjustment, but in terms of a damaging assault on traditional networks of obligation and exchange between groups (including between "wife-givers" and "wife-takers" and the living and dead) that can perpetuate distress if unresolved.

(Footnote 22 continued)

acknowledge, is surely complicated by the growing recognition that trauma may itself be critically implicated in the genesis of the psychotic-reaction (see Sect. 2.2.1).

[23]Grossly disorganised speech and behaviour denoting psychosis was uniformly picked up by the community-identified arm of our study, whereas no cases of PTSD and only two primary cases of depression were identified this way, suggesting the latter responses to trauma, loss and adversity were not traditionally seen as illnesses. Indeed of the two cases of depression, one clearly had psychotic-depression and the other had concurrent panic-attacks that had included an episode of dramatic fainting (described as *mate kik*—Tetum lit. "little death") that would have made her distress more salient to the community, and precipitated a search for extra-mundane causes.

[24]It is probable that the number of individuals afflicted with PTSD-like symptoms has fallen over time (at least prior to the outbreak of widespread internal violence in 2006). For example, it has been previously proposed by Silove (2007) that PTSD symptoms may reflect an emergency attentional and physiological survival response to threat such that in the years following the humanitarian tragedy in 1999 (and before the internal crisis of 2006–2008), a growing confidence in national security against outside foreign threats may have led to increased natural symptom resolution of trauma related distress (cf. Silove and Steel 2006). This was also at a time when the UN and NGO development presence remained prominent, and hope for future prosperity, even if not currently realised, remained high.

Such cultural understandings and expectations of exchange constitute the fabric of society and are felt to ensure the continued "flow of life" in Timor-Leste.

What predisposes a particular individual to *react* to trauma in one clinical direction as opposed to another is of course multifactorial and difficult to predict prospectively. However the multiplicity and severity of the convergent risk factors for dissociation outlined above might be predicted to lead to greater-mental fragmentation and as such be phenomenologically closer to presentations of psychosis (Sect. 2.2.1) as opposed to more organised dissociative-responses, like dissociative identity disorder (DID; Sect. 3.2), although organising factors may still be at play (see Sects. 4.2 and 5.2).

While the relationship between culturally-sanctioned, and arguably adaptive dissociative-states (such as trance) and "pathological dissociation" remains contested (Kirmayer 1994, 2011; Nijenhuis and van der Hart 2011; van der Hart et al. 2004), Kirmayer (2011, 466) has persuasively argued that culturally-sanctioned "milder forms of dissociation…may be part of a trajectory leading toward the more dramatic [potentially pathological] forms." Following this, we shall propose overlapping models of brief psychotic-like symptoms as described in Timor-Leste. We begin with the *linear* model of traumatic dissociation, but here extended to include an understanding of how traumatic events may become symbolically encoded, such that both personal and cultural symbols may serve as triggers of trauma-related dissociated states of mind, mirroring psychosis, in the context of Timorese practice and belief (see Chap. 2). We will then go on to explore, through a psychoanalytic lens, how internal conflict and phantasy, shape responses to external adversity (Chap. 3) and how the recursive interaction of cultural factors, governing meaning, narrative formation, communication and social roles, may interact with this process (Chap. 4). In particular we will explore how these sociocultural factors, alongside material necessity, may have an organising function, and serve to delimit the expression of distress and functional impairment, in a way that might be seen to confer at least partial adaption and resilience in the face of overwhelming, mentally fragmenting experience. We will also hypothesize how such individual experience and behaviour may, at a higher level of analysis, be seen to confer a cultural revitalising function (Sect. 4.2.3). These models are presented as *ideal types* illustrative of the tension between agentic ("bottom-up") and deterministic ("top-down") accounts of individual and collective responses to trauma; the reality is of course more messy and interactive (see Sect. 1.7.1). Since this model rests on an assumption of dissociation as a model for psychosis, we will explore the foundations for this assumption in depth (Sects. 2.2.1 and 5.1).

1.7 Epistemological Tensions

1.7.1 Pragmatic Tensions

In terms of the research process we need to highlight the practical as well as the epistemological challenges of cross-cultural research with transiently psychotic persons. When unwell, such individuals can be hard to locate and when recovered, a tendency to disavow the experience, particularly for the BRR research cohort, limits access to first person accounts and reflection on experience (cf. Guinness 1992a). While we were able to supplement our understanding with family and key consultant interviews, ethnography, and accounts from non-psychotically traumatised persons, as Hollan (2012) points out, what looks superficially similar as a *cultural category* (e.g. *fulan lotuk*), may belie critical differences in context, causality, agency and experience—something which we endeavour to at least partially respond to in our multilevel model of psychotic-symptoms, and contextualised systemic formulations.

While our reliance on collateral accounts from family members in relation to psychotically unwell individuals, might also have been subject to recall bias in relation to illness episodes attributed to the time of the *fulan lotuk*, the profound darkness manifest in areas with no nocturnal electric lighting at the time of the new moon (which at the time of our study included even the capital, Dili), also ensures such times are notable (and such darkness has further relevance to its symbolic significance—see Sects. 2.3.4 and 3.1.2). However, as Csordas et al. (2010) note, despite cultural issues with the SCID (and perhaps structured-interviews in general), one of the advantages of using it is its ability to anchor and connect events in temporal sequence through systematic enquiry, thereby further reducing the likelihood of erroneous associations. We would argue however that even in the presence of occasional recall bias, the ongoing co-construction of cultural categories, like the *fulan lotuk,* then provides a cultural context for potentially ill persons to "act into" (cf. Pearce 2007) and provides a means through which personal and social meanings might be negotiated by, or on behalf of, psychotically afflicted individuals.

Of course, the use of the SCID, essentially a re-working of DSM-IV in a structured interview format, is not without problems. Attempts to apply the assumptions of a Western illness model, encoded in the SCID, during the interviews appeared, as others have found (Csordas et al. 2010), stifling and frustrating to interviewees whose explanatory models, illness narratives and even underlying illness experience were often at odds with this framework.[25] Of course this may also partly reflect cultural unfamiliarity with structured interviews, which may contravene usual styles of social relating and narrating. Indeed even the looser structure of the SEMI appeared inhibitory and restricting at times, to both participants and interviewers alike, and our richest qualitative data came from the more open-ended, fluid conversations, which preceded more formal clinical assessment. The generation of richer illness narratives in this manner also allowed greater confidence in the accuracy and authenticity of informants' responses through minimising suggestion or "demand characteristics" of more structured

[25]Kleinman (1987) warned such universalising assumption may constitute a "category fallacy", with the consequent potential to simply *reproduce* rather than *revise* existing Euro-American illness categories and assumptions (Barrett 2004).

psychometric interviews (cf. Kagee 2004; see Sect. 1.6) that may have compromised the findings of earlier studies (e.g. Modvig et al. 2000). Csordas (2010) reminds us however that our sociocultural positioning as doctors would be as likely to have shaped responses as much as the questions themselves.

Nonetheless, while our findings from the SCID verses our more qualitatively focused interview techniques, certainly have the potential to confuse and contradict, they might also be seen as providing complimentary perspectives that are particularly pertinent to the kind of multi-systemic account we are seeking (Csordas et al. 2010). Indeed we would contend, in the absence of full ethnographic participant–observation, that our movement from unstructured narrative, to semi-structured interview, to the more structured approach of the SCID, not only increased flow and yield, but hopefully also the overall validity of our findings (see Sect. 1.2).

1.7.2 Theoretical Tensions

Any contemporary account of mental illness in the Global South must grapple with questions of epistemology, the most salient tension being that between deterministic and agentic accounts of the human condition. Within transcultural psychiatric research and practice these are well illustrated by the various, overlapping rather than synonymous, conceptual antagonisms: *positivism* versus *constructivism* (Gaines 1992); *naturalistic* versus *personalistic* (Littlewood 1996); *natural kinds* versus *human kinds* (Hacking 1999); *etic* versus *emic* approaches (Headland et al. 1990); and *evidence base medicine* versus *cultural competence* (Kirmayer 2012). Following Gone and Kirmayer (2010) we endorse Hacking's (1999) notion of "interactive kinds" which is implicit in the work presented here. Hacking proposed that the very concepts, categories and/or classifications used to describe *self-aware* human subjects in likelihood changes the nature of what is being experienced and observed by others, through a recursive "looping" process. This is not simply a passive deterministic process, but requires an active interaction between apparently determined facts and events pertaining to the human condition ("natural kinds") and the human constructions of these facts and events ("human kinds).[26]

Another helpful model for considering this interaction between determinism and agency is the so called Cambridge Model developed by Berrios (2014a, b). In this model whether on account of a biological insult or semantic dissonance (which can

---

[26]Hacking (1999) initially approaches the problem appearing to assume that although interactive effects occur, that may change both the inner experience and outward manifestation of human *natural kinds*, the actual nature of these kinds remains unchanged. However he tentatively concludes, at least for mental illness, that in so far as looping effects must ultimately be reflected in brain circuits, the very neurobiological nature of phenomena under study, might also shift correspondingly through this process over time. This concept of "biolooping" (Hacking 1999, 123) has been taken up by critical and cultural neuroscientists as a core critique of theories of neuroscientific reductionism (Choudhury and Slaby 2012).

clearly be extended to the psychological impact of social adversity and/or interpersonal trauma—see Sects. 4.1 and 5.3—Fig. 5.1b) the self is threatened by inchoate experience and seeks to find a resolution. The attempted resolution is an act of agency in which the individual attempts to give this inchoate experience some form and expression, essentially though personal, familial or cultural "configurators"—in essence symbols. Berrios proposes that such symbols serves both intrapsychic and socially expressive/performative functions and as such this model is compatible with the ideas of Victor Turner and Garneth Obeyesekere whom we have drawn upon in this work (see Sects. 3.1.2, 3.1.4 and 4.2.1). Berrios (2014a, 68, Endnote 20) acknowledges a person's choice of configurators in "automatic" but defers the question of whether the choice is consciously or unconsciously made, and never really develops an account of what individual and sociocultural factors influence configurator choice. This requires an account of both unconscious motivation and symbol formation (see Sect. 3.1), alongside an understanding of how symbols bridge the personal and the social (see Sects. 3.1.4 and 4.2.1), that we will discuss in the ensuing chapters.

Implicit in our work is also a negotiated understanding of agency, that expresses itself at multiple levels, but finds its limits in deterministic exigencies, whether these be rooted in the body, socioeconomic privations or deprivations, or cultural and political barriers.[27] This interplay between agency and determinism is as pertinent to the study of psychosis as of other manifestations of mental distress (Hopper 2008). In this work, we also attempt to respond to the call to offer up whole system descriptions relating to individual mental states and behaviour. This goes hand-in-hand with the related call for "epistemic pluralism" (Kirmayer 2012; Hinton and Kirmayer 2013; de Jong and Reis 2013). This is reflected in our multi-layered methodology and use of secondary sources—the former moving from narrative evocation, to semi-structured, to structured interview; the latter ranging from neuroscience to historical and economic-political analysis. The difficulty, however, is in integrating such a range of data and models, within an overarching synthesis. Papers and collected volumes continue to proliferate attempting to address the vexed questions of causality and ontology in psychiatry, but no consensus appears likely anytime soon.

Different levels of explanation are generally acknowledged, but attempted syntheses range from the reductionist idea that such models represent different vantage points on the same underlying neural process, to concepts of hierarchical influence (Murphy 2008); although the direction of influence is itself often contested (which has the stronger influence, genes or social context?), and in fact, as Burnham and Harris have summarised (1995) from a comparable perspective, *different contexts may be hierarchically privileged at different times*. Interactive models, including

[27]The acknowledgement of both agency and its limits, conceptualized as "situated freedom" (Lopez and Willis 2004, 729), has been central to the project of interpretive phenomenology. This tension continues to be evoked and, in Rorty's (1989) words, *redescribed* in other disciplines, including anthropology, via cultural phenomenology (Ortner 2006), and narrative/systemic family therapy (Lang and McAdam 1995); both of which have informed the current work.

that of Hacking and Berrios above, are both inclusive and persuasive in this regard. As Kendler (in Kendler and Parnas (eds.) 2008, 100) puts it, "hard reductionism will not work because no one level is the 'fundamental' one. Rather each modifies the other." This would appear to apply equally to social determinism as to biological determinism (cf. Gaines 1991).

While conceptual contradiction can also reflect errors and distortion in both research findings and/or theory, requiring revision,[28] it may also sometimes be apparent rather than real. The constructivist acceptance that models are just that, *models*, that may yield useful answers to specific questions in particular contexts (Hoffman 1990) is therefore refreshingly transparent and applies equally well to the natural sciences.[29] In human contexts, the problem arises however, when different understandings generate apparently incompatible, rather than complimentary, solutions. This may manifest as antagonism between levels of explanation and/or intervention, arising from epistemic pluralism.[30] For example at the level of explanation, in the context of "auditory hallucinations" dealt with in our work (see Sect. 2.2.1), the difference between an approach advocating voice elimination/repression, usually with antipsychotic medication, as opposed to aiming at integration (of voices representing different "split off" self-parts), or else constructive transformation of the person's relationship with their voices (for example, where viewed as spirit allies or ancestors) is hard to reconcile[31] (Rodger 2011 and 2013). It is also becomes a moral issue when psychiatric power limits the choices of services users, albeit with benevolent intent and sometimes unavoidably in its dual-role as agent of social control (Bracken and Thomas 2005; Middleton 2015). An example of antagonism at the level of intervention, would be when a solution of apparent benefit to the individual, may be potentially harmful to others in the wider community; a concern raised when Western models of mental health are exported with little adaption to other cultural contexts, potentially undermining local efficacious beliefs and practices, and catalysing cultural re-configurations of self from

---

[28]Such error is inevitable in an ambitious and multidisciplinary project like our and our theorising will surely generate more questions than answers, to be addressed in more focused research, whether in epidemiology, ethnography, experimental psychology, neuroscience or clinical outcome research.

[29]Such as in *wave* verses *particle* theories of light, which can both give rise to useful predictions, dependent on the question or context.

[30]This may further reflection epistemological tensions between agentic and deterministic understandings, however pragmatism in help-seeking may also supervene (cf. Young 1982). In her earlier focus-groups and survey of community understanding of mental illness in Timor-Leste, Graves (2003) similarly noted that concepts of causality did not necessarily predict expressed perceived treatment options.

[31]"Medication can only be reconciled with the ancestor/spirit metaphor [of voices] as 'something that might take the edge of my distress' while engaging with this process of restitution, although not all voice-hearers find this acceptable or necessary" (Rodger 2011, 430).

the *sociocentric* to the *individualistic*[32] (see also Sect. 1.1, Footnote 5 for citations exploring the cultural impact of psychopharmaceuticals in this domain).

To be further transparent, we should also acknowledge how as researchers, are own theoretical predilections may be reflective of different professional cultures, identities, ideologies, or our own lived experience, as much as genuine scientific commitments or objections, although hopefully these domains are not mutually exclusive. As authors of this work, we have self-consciously aligned ourselves with wider movements within critical psychology and psychiatry, and developed a sensitivity to both trauma and social justice, alongside a recognition of the need for empowerment and recognition of agency—borne out of both personal and professional experience. At the same time, we would argue that models of understanding and practice that marginalise such aspects of experience are incomplete, perpetuate structural violence, and often limit therapeutic progress. Indeed more mainstream research groups, including the Cambridge Group,[33] are now articulating similar concerns and attempting to grapple and bridge the gap between deterministic and agentic accounts of mental illness, including psychosis.

1.7.3 Dialogue with the Global Mental Health Movement

The epistemological tensions described above, account for much of the polarisation of positions seen in response to the call to arms on Global Mental Health (GMH), launched in 2007, to both approbation and dismay, in a special edition of the Lancet (Vol 370(9591)) and built upon in a key paper in Nature linking to wider "Grand Challenges" for global health (Collins et al. 2011). These have been energetically followed-up with a number of further high impact journal special editions, series and sections (Lancet 2011, 378(9801), PLoS Medicine 2009, 6(10)—2010, 7(2) and 2012, 9(5)—2013, 10(4); Harvard Review of Psychiatry 2012, 20(1); International Journal of Epidemiology 2014, 43(2) and stand-alone articles (e.g. Vikram Patel and Saxena 2014).

---

[32]With Halliburton (2004, 86), speaking from a somewhat comparable South Indian context, we acknowledge that "it should not be assumed that there is a clear dichotomy between the sociocentric [Austronesian] and the individualistic westerner or that the [Austronesian] person is wholly socio-centric" and similarly that "There are realms of autonomy in [Austronesian] societies (Ewing 1991) as well as ways in which Americans are sociocentric (Kusserow, 1999)" (95, Endnote 6).

[33]As Berrios (2014a, 32), puts it "a correlation between symptom S and brain site B should no longer be considered as constituting a sufficient ethical warrant for therapeutically intervening on site B. It would also be necessary to know the level of participation of the sufferer in the construction of his complaint" although such participation need not be conscious. He concludes that this would "show that sufferers are far more active and participatory in the formation of their mental symptoms than the current neurobiological model allows" (39). We would extend this point to models of psychological trauma, in so far that trauma wounds, in part, because it violates our agency (further reflected in narrative), and our agency (both conscious and unconscious) also shapes our response (see Sects. 2.3.1 and 4.1, Chap. 3).

While emergent key proposals (e.g. Collins 2011) appear reasonably balanced between attention to biological and sociocultural factors, both as causal risk factors and sites of response, critical commentators have highlighted the gap between the rhetoric and reality, in which treatment has become a proxy for de-contextualised individual medication and/or psychotherapies, and success or failure evaluated only at the individual level, to the neglect of the multiple levels of analysis advocated for by Hinton and Kirmayer (2013) and De Jong and Reis (2013).

The language of diagnosis and disorder also carries with it contested universalising assumptions and downplays resilience. Discrepancies in power between donor and recipient countries, professions and groups, may further give rise to an imbalance in attention to different levels of explanation and intervention described above, and in which individuals and communities are seen as passive victims, rather than active, resourceful survivors—the concern being that local notions and practices underlying resilience will be undermined (Campbell and Burgess 2012; Summerfield 2012). This is of potential concern, given that even in developed country settings, research is emerging suggesting that over reliance on psychopharmaceuticals, may—besides being often at the expense of attention to meaning and contextual factors (Bracken et al. 2012)—contribute to a disempowering "external locus of control" (Harrow and Jobe 2007; see Sect. 5.2.1), and neuroadaptations that in the long-term may foster chronicity (Whitaker 2010) and lead to poorer functional outcomes (Wunderink et al. 2013).

Indeed in this regard, Read (2012) has highlighted that the exportation of psychiatric paradigms and treatment to the low and middle income countries, circumvents the growing critique of Western psychiatric treatment in the West itself (Bracken et al. 2012; Myers 2010; Whitaker 2010). Additionally the lack of regulation, newly targeted marketing, and widespread availability of conventionally prescription-only psychiatric medications, "over the counter," in many low to middle income country settings, further increases the potential for harms described (Fernando 2012, 2014).

Critiques of the use of Western diagnosis in non-Western settings, beyond that of universalising assumptions and neo-colonialism, come back to implicit biological connotations that easily obscure wider socioeconomic antecedents to distress. While this is no different to auto-critiques of Western psychiatry (Rodger et al. 2014), in low income countries—often characterised by abject poverty, more entrenched gender roles, greater civil conflict and political corruption, and vulnerability to more widespread human rights violations—the stakes for practices that further obfuscate these factors is higher still. A critical approach to psychiatric theory and practice in the West therefore go hand in hand with transcultural psychiatric and medical anthropological approaches both of which have long been concerned with the social determinants of health, which both local cultural practice and Western diagnoses can obscure (Littlewood and Lipsedge 1987).

In defence of the GMH project, advocates of allopathic psychiatry continue to assert the universal applicability of diagnostic categories, invoking the familiar form-content argument, and point to the high prevalence rates of disorder in low to middle income countries, based on epidemiological findings, side-stepping critiques of their methodology and validity (Kirmayer and Pedersen 2014). They further point to the abject scarcity of mental health professionals per capita, potentially abusive family and local practices in the aetiology and management of psychotic and other mental health presentations (Maj 2011), and point out that the same social indices of adversity cited above, are in themselves significant risk factors for mental disorder, including psychosis and schizophrenia—while accusing critics of romanticizing such factors to account for purported better outcomes of schizophrenia in developing countries (Burns 2009; Cohen et al. 2007).

Finding much needed middle ground, Campbell and Burgess (2012), point to the strategic use of health-focused discourse: which permits "piggybacking" on existing infrastructures; the need to keep initial messages simple and coherent to build effective alliances; and the requisite to avoid alienating donors and governments early on by talk of radical social and political change. They also challenge notions of passive victimhood, arguing that communities have some agency when choosing to engage with (or resist) external agencies and donors, for their own ends.[34] In this respect, we would also agree that while there are legitimate concerns in relation to Western psychiatric cultural imperialism ("neo-colonisation") (Fernando 2014; Summerfield 2012) and "interpretive violence" (Corin, Rangaswami, and Ramachandran 2004, 110), culture is also essentially dynamic and adaptive—and in a globalised world, cultural identities essentially hybrid, which in turn may create new opportunities for self-identity and social positioning (Corin and Bibeau 2006). In any case, we might note that forces beyond (but inclusive of) psychiatry are already shaping local cultural worlds, in ways that demand change[35] (Kirmayer 2006). Equally however, individuals and cultures can be resilient, in the face of such external forces of change, as we go onto address in our discussion of cultural revitalisation (see Sect. 4.2.3). We also acknowledge here the important healing function an attempted return to traditional cultural identities may have (Gone 2013).

Campbell and Burgess (2012) further note the importance of engaging communities, and creating "safe social spaces" alongside "receptive social environments" (pp. 389–390) in order to tap into, develop and endorse local knowledge, support networks and practices, while aspiring towards political engagement. Finally where abusive practices, such as shackling, do exist, they note these are often linked to unimaginable social and economic contexts of survival beyond health that limit management options, and they endorse the need for partnership and collaboration,[36] rather than high-ground moralising.

---

[34]However they note this would be considerably facilitated by agencies aspiring towards co-creating Habermas' "idealized notion of the 'public sphere', where equal respect and recognition to the views of all participants irrespective of their social status and institutional power" (Campbell and Burgess 2012, 389).

[35]Although acknowledging this, we should not forget, that the medicalisation and contingent de-politicisation of such change, is an extremely potent, undercover weapon, capable of serving a neo-liberal agenda.

[36]Within our own study we strove to build partnerships with government, community leaders, local NGOs, and our Timorese colleagues, validating their expert local knowledge as "culture

While our study focused on clinical assessment, explanatory models and cultural illness narratives, rather than intervention (although we referred people on to other agencies where needed), it is important to explicitly acknowledge that how mental distress is framed will have critical implications for both community response and therapeutic intervention. Our diagnostic formulation, using the rather generic category of PDNOS, while clinically justified, also carries the strategic advantage of implying "mental and behavioural phenomena poorly captured by existing concepts and opening up the way for debate about their qualities" (see Sect. 1.5.1), hopefully less skewed by dominant biological constructs.

While local solutions should be encouraged, sought out and endorsed, we recognise that we should not necessarily denigrate or exclude our own contributions to understanding complex patterns of behaviour in other cultures (which can be the flipside to the equally unhelpful "exotification of the other"). Exceptionally this may even involve taking a position against a particular local cultural practice (e.g. witchcraft accusations targeting children (Reis 2013) see Sect. 1.1, Footnote 5). While such a position, alongside particular epistemic frames (such as psychoanalytic theorising), appear, as Byron Good (2012, 32) points out, to potentially involve the uncomfortable, indeed untenable, position, reminiscent of "colonial anthropology of 'knowing better' than those with whom we work"; as he further elaborates this should involve "not only a different form of theorising, but a different form of listening and engagement that involves a mode of *mutual discovery*" [emphasis added] with "interpretations of these matters always provisional, open to revision."

Nonetheless we need to be clear, this work is not intended to directly influence the beliefs and practices of local people in Timor-Leste, but rather through the multiple lenses of anthropology, trauma theory and psychoanalysis, to support our own understanding, and that of other "Western" oriented clinicians and researchers —and this includes an acknowledgement and admiration of the psychological "work of culture" already being done (cf. Obeyesekere 1990). We would assert that frequently symbolic cultural forms and practices may capture (and indeed transform) emotional, relational and even political dilemmas (Traube 2007; cf. Chen 2004), for both individual and group as, or more effectively (and in healing terms, efficaciously—see Sects. 3.1.2, 4.1.1 and 4.2; cf. Kirmayer 1993), than any imported theories and practices that lack resonance with local knowledge and ways of seeing.

In this respect, while a dialogue of our results and reflections with Timorese government and community leaders on the ground remains important, the community of practice that this book is more specifically aimed at is Western aid agencies, international public health workers, and local practitioners already deploying an imported Western model of mental health and intervention, and

(Footnote 36 continued)

brokers" but exchanging it with training in our own and the development of transferable research skills alongside respectful remuneration policies for their services.

indeed academic theorists and practitioners of the Western model *in any context,* to promote a greater reticence and respect for sociocultural complexity to inform understanding and intervention.

As Silove and Ward (2014) note "a key criticism of the GMH movement is that it has blinded itself to the complexity of culture in its haste to roll out packaged programmes of care in low-income and middle-income countries"—a criticism of culture, similar to that made of the WHO studies into cross-national long-term outcomes of schizophrenia (Hopper 2004). While our own study was not of ethnographic depth, through existing ethnography, the use of local cultural consultants and that unfolding in individual and family interviews, we have sought to incorporate a concept of culture that is at once, both general (and potentially transferable) and specific, shedding light on how culture may shape illness, in addition to how illness may in turn shed light on culture.

We privilege no particular solution, but endorse a utilitarian *sociopolitical* understanding of mental distress and intervention (Kupfer et al. 2002), in which the relative merits of medical, psychological, educational, economic, religious and other cultural understandings and interventions are judged on their relative merits, providing analyses of outcome are at the multiples levels, beyond the individual, described. As Kirmayer (2012, 252) notes, "CC [cultural competence] needs research to validate its practices. EBP [evidence based-practice] needs CC to determine the generalizability of its knowledge into local appropriate interventions." We will always be behind such an understanding, and the immediacy of suffering may force our hand to act (Kirmayer 2012) but at least we should aspire to approach this ideal.

References

American Psychiatric Association (APA). 2000. *Diagnostic and statistical manual of mental disorders*, 4th ed., Text Rev. Washington, DC: Author.: American Psychiatric Publishing.

American Psychiatric Association (APA). 2013. *Diagnostic and statistical manual of mental disorders*, 5th ed. Washington, D.C: Washington, DC: Author.

Barrett, Robert J. 2004. Kurt Schneider in Borneo: Do first rank symptoms apply to the Iban? In *Schizophrenia, culture, and subjectivity: The edge of experience*, eds. Janis Hunter Jenkins, and Robert J. Barrett, 87–109. Cambridge, UK: Cambridge University Press.

Bellwood, Peter, James Fox, and Darrell Tryon, eds. 1995. *The Austronesians: Historical and comparative perspectives*. Canberra, ACT, Australia: ANU E Press. EPUB file. http://epress.anu.edu.au/titles/comparative-austronesian-series/austronesians_citation/pdf-download.

Benamer, Sarah, ed. 2010. *Telling stories?: Attachment based approach to the treatment of psychosis*. Karnac Books.

Berrios, German E. 2014a. History and epistemology of psychopathology. In *Philosophical issues in psychiatry III: The nature and sources of historical change*, eds. Kenneth S. Kendler, and Josef Parnas, 30–50. Oxford, UK: Oxford University Press. EPUB file.

Berrios, German E. 2014b. The role of cultural configurators in the formation of mental symptoms. In *Philosophical issues in psychiatry III: The nature and sources of historical change*, eds. Kenneth S. Kendler, and Josef Parnas, 107–115. Oxford, UK: Oxford University Press. EPUB file.

Bibeau, Gilles. 1997. Cultural psychiatry in a creolizing world: Questions for a new research agenda. *Transcultural Psychiatry* 34(1): 9–41. doi:10.1177/136346159703400102.

Bovensiepen, Judith. 2009. Spiritual landscapes of life and death in the central highlands of East Timor. *Anthropological Forum* 19: 323–338.

Bracken, Pat. 2001. Post-modernity and post-traumatic stress disorder. *Social Science and Medicine* 53(6): 733–743.

Bracken, Pat, J.E. Giller, and D. Summerfield. 1995. Psychological responses to war and atrocity: The limitations of current concepts. *Social Science and Medicine* 40(8): 1073–1082.

Bracken, Patrick, and Philip Thomas. 2005. *Postpsychiatry: Mental health in a postmodern world.* Oxford: Oxford University Press.

Bracken, Pat, Philip Thomas, Sami Timimi, Eia Asen, Graham Behr, Carl Beuster, Seth Bhunnoo, et al. 2012. Psychiatry beyond the current paradigm. *The British Journal of Psychiatry* 201(6): 430–434. doi:10.1192/bjp.bp.112.109447.

Burnham, John, and Queenie Harris. 1995. Emerging ethnicity—A tale of three cultures. In *Meeting the Needs of Ethnic Minority Children: Including Refugee, Black and Mixed Parentage Children: A Hanbook for Professionals*, 2nd ed., eds. Kedar Nath Dwivedi, and Ved P. Varma. London: Jessica Kingsley Publishers.

Burns, J. 2009. Dispelling a myth: Developing world poverty, inequality, violence and social fragmentation are not good for outcome in schizophrenia. *African Journal of Psychiatry* 12(3). doi:10.4314/ajpsy.v12i3.48494.

Campbell, C., and R. Burgess. 2012. The role of communities in advancing the goals of the movement for global mental health. *Transcultural Psychiatry* 49(3–4): 379–395. doi:10.1177/1363461512454643.

Carey, Peter. 1999. The Catholic church, religious revival, and the nationalist movement in East Timor, 1975–98. *Indonesia and the Malay World* 27(78): 77. doi:10.1080/13639819908729935.

Carlson, Gabrielle A. 2005. Early onset bipolar disorder: Clinical and research considerations. *Journal of Clinical Child & Adolescent Psychology* 34(2): 333–343. doi:10.1207/s15374424jccp3402_13.

Castagnini, Augusto C. 2010. Wimmer's concept of psychogenic psychosis revisited. *History of Psychiatry* 21(1): 54–66. doi:10.1177/0957154X09338086.

Castagnini, Augusto, and German E. Berrios. 2011. The relationship of acute transient psychoses and schizophrenia. In *Handbook of schizophrenia spectrum disorders*, vol. II, ed. Michael Ritsner, 367–387. Netherlands: Springer.

Castillo, Richard J. 1994a. Spirit possession in south asia, dissociation or hysteria? Part 1: Theoretical background. *Culture, Medicine and Psychiatry* 18(1): 1–21. doi:10.1007/BF01384875.

Castillo, Richard J. 1994b. Spirit possession in south asia, dissociation or hysteria? Part 2: Case histories. *Culture, Medicine and Psychiatry* 18(2): 141–162. doi:10.1007/BF01379447.

Castillo, Richard J. 2006. Effects of culture on recovery from transient psychosis—Psychiatric times' 23(14). http://www.psychiatrictimes.com/display/article/10168/51596.

Chen, Victoria. 2004. The possibility of critical dialogue in the theory of CMM. *Human Systems: The Journal of Systemic Consultation & Management* 15(3): 179–192.

Choudhury, Suparna, and Jan Slaby. 2012. Introduction: Critical neuroscience—Between Lifeworld and Laboratory. In *Critical neuroscience: A handbook of the social and cultural contexts of neuroscience*, eds. Suparna Choudhury, and Jan Slaby, 1–26. Chichester, West Sussex: Wiley-Blackwell.

Cohen, A., V. Patel, R. Thara, and O. Gureje. 2007. Questioning an axiom: Better prognosis for schizophrenia in the developing world? *Schizophrenia Bulletin* 34(2): 229–244. doi:10.1093/schbul/sbm105.

Collins, Pamela Y., Vikram Patel, Sarah S. Joestl, Dana March, Thomas R. Insel, and Abdallah S. Daar. 2011. Grand challenges in global mental health. *Nature* 475(7354): 27–30. doi:10.1038/475027a.

Cooper, Rachel. 2004. What is wrong with the DSM? *History of Psychiatry* 15(1): 5–25. doi:10.1177/0957154X04039343.

Corin, Ellen, and Gilles Bibeau. 2006. Speaking about culture in multiple voices. *Transcultural Psychiatry* 43(1): 106–125. doi:10.1177/1363461506061760.

Corin, Ellen, Thara Rangaswami, and Padmavati Ramachandran. 2004. Living through a staggering world: The play of signifiers in early psychosis in South India. In *Schizophrenia, culture, and subjectivity: The edge of experience*, eds. Janis Hunter Jenkins, and Robert J. Barrett, 110–45. Cambridge, UK: Cambridge University Press.

Csordas, Thomas J., Christopher Dole, Allen Tran, Matthew Strickland, and Michael G. Storck. 2010. Ways of asking, ways of telling: A methodological comparison of ethnographic and research diagnostic interviews. *Culture, Medicine and Psychiatry* 34(1): 29–55. doi:10.1007/s11013-009-9160-4.

Cutajar, Margaret C., Paul E. Mullen, James R.P. Ogloff, Stuart D. Thomas, David L. Wells, and Josie Spataro. 2010. Schizophrenia and other psychotic disorders in a cohort of sexually abused children. *Archives of General Psychiatry* 67(11): 1114–1119. doi:10.1001/archgenpsychiatry.2010.147.

de Jong, Joop T., and Ria Reis. 2013. Collective trauma processing: Dissociation as a way of processing postwar traumatic stress in Guinea Bissau. *Transcultural Psychiatry* 50(5): 644–661. doi:10.1177/1363461513500517.

Desjarlais, Robert. 2012. Commentary: Redescriptions. *Ethos* 40(1): 97–103. doi:10.1111/j.1548-1352.2011.01233.x.

Durand, F. 2009. Recurring crises in Timor-Leste failed state or country in search of a project? *Lusotopie* 16(2): 65–81.

Elsass, P. 2001. Individual and collective traumatic memories: A qualitative study of post-traumatic stress disorder symptoms in two Latin American Localities. *Transcultural Psychiatry* 38(3): 306.

Faergeman, Poul M. 1963. *Psychogenic psychoses. A description and follow-up of psychoses following psychological stress*, 1st ed. Butterworths

Farram, Steven. 2010. *A political history of West Timor: 1901–1967*. LAP Lambert Academic Publishing.

Fernandez, J.W. 1978. African religious movements. *Annual Review of Anthropology* 7(1): 195–234. doi:10.1146/annurev.an.07.100178.001211.

Fernando, Suman. 2014. *Mental health worldwide: Culture, globalization and development*. UK: Palgrave Macmillan.

Fernando, Suman. 2012. Challenges for mental health development in low- and middle-income countries. Presented at the Advanced Study Institute, McGill University. https://vimeo.com/48900799.

First, Michael B., Robert L. Spitzer, Miriam Gibbon, and Janet B.W. Williams. 2002. *Structured clinical interview for DSM-IV-TR axis I disorders, research version, non-patient edition. (SCID-I/NP)*. New York: Biometrics Research, New York State Psychiatric Institute.

Fonagy, Peter, Gyorgy Gergely, Elliot Jurist, and Mary Target. 2002. *Affect regulation, mentalization, and the development of the self*. New York: Other Press.

Fonagy, Peter, George Gergely, and Mary Target. 2008. Psychoanalytic constructs and attachment theory. In *Handbook of attachment*, 2nd ed., eds. Jude Cassidy, and Phillip R. Shaver, 783–810. New York, NY: Guilford Press.

Forman, S. 1977. 'East Timor: Exchange and political hierarchy at the time of the European discoveries. In *Economic exchange and social interaction in Southeast Asia: Perspectives from prehistory, history and ethnography*. ed. Karl Hutterer, 97–112. Ann Arbor: Centre for South and Southeast Asian Studies, University of Michigan.

Fox, James J. 1996. The paradox of powerlessness: Timor in historical perspective. Presented at The Nobel Peace Prize Symposium: Focus on East Timor, University of Oslo, December 9. https://digitalcollections.anu.edu.au/bitstream/1885/41370/3/TimorOslo_Paper.pdf.

Gaines, Atwood D. 1991. Cultural constructivism: Sickness histories and the understanding of ethnomedicines beyond critical medical anthropologies. In *Anthropologies of medicine*, eds.

Beatrix Pfleiderer, and Gilles Bibeau, 221–58. Vieweg+Teubner Verlag. http://link.springer.com/chapter/10.1007/978-3-322-87859-5_17.

Gaines, Atwood D. 1992. From DSM-I to III-R; voices of self, mastery and the other: A cultural constructivist reading of U.S. psychiatric classification. *Social Science & Medicine* 35(1): 3–24 (1982).

Ganguli, Mary, Graham Ratcliff, Vijay Chandra, Sujatha Sharma, Joanne Gilby, Rajesh Pandav, Steven Belle, et al. 1995. A hindi version of the MMSE: The development of a cognitive screening instrument for a largely illiterate rural elderly population in India. *International Journal of Geriatric Psychiatry* 10(5): 367–377. doi:10.1002/gps.930100505.

Gergely, György, and John S. Watson. 1999. Early socio-emotional development: Contingency perception and the social-biofeedback model. In *Early Social Cognition: Understanding Others in the First Months of Life*, ed. Philippe Rochat, 101–36. Hillsdale, NJ: Lawrence Erlbaum Associates.

Gone, Joseph P. 2013. Redressing first nations historical trauma: Theorizing mechanisms for indigenous culture as mental health treatment. *Transcultural Psychiatry* 50(5): 683–706. doi:10.1177/1363461513487669.

Gone, Joseph P., and Laurence J. Kirmayer. 2010. On the wisdom of considering culture and context in psychopathology. In *Contemporary Directions in Psychopathology: Scientific Foundations of the DSM-V and ICD-11*, eds. Theodore Millon, Robert F. Krueger and Erik Simonsen, 72–96. New York, NY: Guildford Press.

Good, Byron J. 2012. Phenomenology, psychoanalysis, and subjectivity in Java. *Ethos* 40(1): 24–36. doi:10.1111/j.1548-1352.2011.01229.x.

Good, Byron J. 2004. Experiences of psychosis in Javanese culture: Reflections on a case of acute, recurrent psychosis in contemporary Yogyakarta, Indonesia. In *Schizophrenia, culture, and subjectivity: The edge of experience*, eds. Janis Hunter Jenkins, and Robert J. Barrett, 167–95. Cambridge, UK: Cambridge University Press.

Graves, Jenni. 2003. Knowledge, attitudes and responses to mental illness. Democratic Republic of East Timor: East Timor National Mental Health Project, Ministry of Health.

Guinness, E.A. 1992a. Brief reactive psychosis and the major functional psychoses: Descriptive case studies in Africa. *The British Journal of Psychiatry. Supplement* 16: 24–41.

Guinness, E A. 1992b. Relationship between the neuroses and brief reactive psychosis: Descriptive case studies in Africa. *The British Journal of Psychiatry. Supplement* 16:12–23.

Gunn, Geoffrey C. 2001. The five hundred years Timorese Funu. In *Bitter flowers, sweet flowers: East Timor, Indonesia, and the world community*, eds. Richard Tanter, Mark Selden, and Stephen Rosskamm Shalom, 3–14. Lanham, Maryland: Rowman & Littlefield.

Hacking, Ian. 1999. *The social construction of what?* Harvard: Harvard University Press.

Halliburton, Murphy. 2004. Finding a fit: Psychiatric pluralism in South India and its implications for WHO studies of mental disorder. *Transcultural Psychiatry* 41(1): 80–98. doi:10.1177/1363461504041355.

Harrow, Martin, and Thomas H. Jobe. 2007. Factors involved in outcome and recovery in schizophrenia patients not on antipsychotic medications: A 15-year multifollow-up study. *The Journal of Nervous and Mental Disease* 195(5): 406–414. doi:10.1097/01.nmd.0000253783.32338.6e.

Hatta, S.M. 1996. A Malay crosscultural worldview and forensic review of Amok. *Australasian Psychiatry* 30(4): 505–510.

Headland, Thomas N., Kenneth L. Pike, and Marvin Harris, eds. 1990. *Emics and etics: The insider/outsider debate. Frontiers of Anthropology* (Vol. 7). Thousand Oaks, CA, US: Sage Publications, Inc.

Hicks, David. 2004. *Tetum ghosts & kin: Fertility and gender in East Timor*, 2nd ed. Waveland Pr Inc.

Hinton, D.E., and L.J. Kirmayer. 2013. Local responses to trauma: Symptom, affect, and healing. *Transcultural Psychiatry* 50(5): 607–621. doi:10.1177/1363461513506529.

Hoffman, Lynn. 1990. Constructing realities: An art of lenses. *Family Process* 29(1): 1–12. doi:10.1111/j.1545-5300.1990.00001.x.

Hollan, Douglas. 2012. On the varieties and particularities of cultural experience. *Ethos* 40(1): 37–53. doi:10.1111/j.1548-1352.2011.01230.x.
Hollender, Marc H., and Steven J. Hirsch. 1964. Hysterical psychosis. *American Journal of Psychiatry* 120(11): 1066–1074. doi:10.1176/appi.ajp.120.11.1066.
Holmes, Jeremy. 2001. *The search for the secure base: Attachment theory and psychotherapy*. Hove, East Sussex: Psychology Press.
Hopper, Kim. 1991. Some old questions for the new cross-cultural psychiatry. *Medical Anthropology Quarterly, New Series* 5(4): 299–330.
Hopper, Kim. 2004. Interrogating the meaning of "culture" in the WHO international studies of schizophrenia. In *Schizophrenia, culture, and subjectivity: The edge of experience*, eds. Janis Hunter Jenkins, and Robert J. Barrett, 62–86. Cambridge, UK: Cambridge University Press.
Hopper, Kim. 2008. Outcomes elsewhere: Course of psychosis in "other cultures". In *Society and psychosis*, eds. Craig Morgan, Kwame McKenzie, and Paul Fearon, 198–216. Cambridge: Cambridge University Press.
Hopper, Kim, Glynn Harrison, Aleksandar Janca, and Norman Sartorius, eds. 2007. *Recovery from schizophrenia: An international perspective : A report from the WHO collaborative project, the international study of schizophrenia*. Oxford: Oxford University Press.
Hoshmand, Lisa Tsoi. 2007. Cultural-ecological perspectives on the understanding and assessment of trauma. In *Cross-cultural assessment of psychological trauma and PTSD*, eds. John P. Wilson, and Catherine So-kum Tang, 31–50. International and Cultural Psychology Series, Part 2. Boston, MA: Springer.
Jackson, Murray, and Paul Williams. 1994. *Unimaginable storms: A search for meaning in psychosis*. Karnac Books.
Jadhav, S., M.G. Weiss, and R. Littlewood. 2001. Cultural experience of depression among White Britons in London. *Anthropology & Medicine* 8(1): 47–69.
Janca, A., M. Kastrup, H. Katschnig, J.J. Lopez-Ibor, J.E. Mezzich, and N. Sartorius. 1996. The world health organization short disability assessment schedule (WHO DAS-S): A tool for the assessment of difficulties in selected areas of functioning of patients with mental disorders. *Social Psychiatry and Psychiatric Epidemiology* 31(6): 349–354. doi:10.1007/BF00783424.
Jauch, D.A., and W.T. Carpenter. 1988. Reactive psychosis. II. Does DSM-III-R define a third psychosis? *The Journal of Nervous and Mental Disease* 176(2): 82–86.
Jenkins, Janis H. 2011. *Pharmaceutical self: The global shaping of experience in an age of psychopharmacology*, 1st ed. Santa Fe, N.M: SAR Press.
Jenkins, Janis Hunter, and Robert J. Barrett (eds.). 2004. *Schizophrenia, culture, and subjectivity: The edge of experience*. Cambridge, UK: Cambridge University Press.
Jilek, W.G., and L. Jilek-Aall. 1970. Transient psychoses in Africans. *Psychopathology* 3(6): 337–364.
Kagee, Ashraf. 2004. Do South African former detainees experience post-traumatic stress? Circumventing the demand characteristics of psychological assessment. *Transcultural Psychiatry* 41(3): 323–336.
Kendler, Kenneth S., and Josef Parnas, eds. 2008. *Philosophical issues in psychiatry: Explanation, phenomenology, and nosology*. Johns Hopkins University Press.
Kessler, Ronald C. 2000. Posttraumatic stress disorder: The burden to the individual and to society. *The Journal of Clinical Psychiatry* 61(Suppl 5): 4–12; discussion 13–14.
Kessler, Ronald C., D.R. Rubinow, C. Holmes, J.M. Abelson, and S. Zhao. 1997. The epidemiology of DSM-III-R bipolar I disorder in a general population survey. *Psychological Medicine* 27(05): 1079–1089.
Kessler, Ronald C., Wai Tat Chiu, Olga Demler, Kathleen R. Merikangas, and Ellen E. Walters. 2005. Prevalence, severity, and comorbidity of 12-Month DSM-IV disorders in the national comorbidity survey replication. *Archives of General Psychiatry* 62(6): 617–627. doi:10.1001/archpsyc.62.6.617.
Kingsbury, Damien. 2010. National identity in Timor-Leste: Challenges and opportunities. *South East Asia Research* 18(1): 133–159. doi:10.5367/000000010790959820.

Kirmayer, Laurence J. 1993. Healing and the invention of metaphor: The effectiveness of symbols revisited. *Culture, Medicine and Psychiatry* 17(2): 161–195. doi:10.1007/BF01379325.

Kirmayer, Laurence J. 1996. Confusion of the senses: Implications of ethnocultural variations in somatoform and dissociative disorders for PTSD. In *Ethnocultural aspects of posttraumatic stress disorder: Issues, research, and clinical applications*, eds. Anthony J. Marsella, Matthew J. Friedman, Ellen T. Gerrity, and Raymond M. Scurfield, 131–163. Washington, DC: American Psychological Association.

Kirmayer, Laurence J. 2006. Beyond the "new cross-cultural psychiatry": Cultural biology, discursive psychology and the ironies of globalization. *Transcultural Psychiatry* 43(1): 126–144. doi:10.1177/1363461506061761.

Kirmayer, Laurence J. 2011. Defining and delimiting trauma-related dissociation: A view from cultural psychiatry. *Journal of Trauma & Dissociation* 12(4): 465–468. doi:10.1080/15299732.2011.570235.

Kirmayer, Laurence J. 2012. Cultural competence and evidence-based practice in mental health: Epistemic communities and the politics of pluralism. *Social Science and Medicine* 75(2): 249–256. doi:10.1016/j.socscimed.2012.03.018.

Kirmayer, Laurence J. 1994. Pacing the void: Social and cultural dimensions of dissociation. In *Dissociation: Culture, mind, and body*, ed. David Spiegel, 91–122

Kirmayer, Laurence J., and Daina M. Sc Crafa. 2014. What kind of science for psychiatry?' *Frontiers in Human Neuroscience* 8:435. doi:10.3389/fnhum.2014.00435.

Kirmayer, Laurence J., and Duncan Pedersen. 2014. Toward a New Architecture for Global Mental Health. *Transcultural Psychiatry* 51(6): 759–776. doi:10.1177/1363461514557202.

Kleinman, Arthur. 1978. Concepts and a model for the comparison of medical systems as cultural systems. *Social Science & Medicine Part B: Medical Anthropology* 12: 85–93.

Kleinman, A. 1987. Anthropology and psychiatry. The role of culture in cross-cultural research on illness. *The British Journal of Psychiatry* 151(4): 447–454. doi:10.1192/bjp.151.4.447.

Kleinman, Arthur. 1988. *The illness narratives: Suffering, healing, and the human condition*. Basic Books.

Kon, Y. 1994. Amok. *The British Journal of Psychiatry* 165(5): 685.

Kupfer, David J., Michael B. First, and Darrel A. Regier (eds.). 2002. *A research agenda for DSM-V*. Washington, DC: American Psychiatric Association.

Lambek, Michael. 2003. Fantasy in practice: Projection and introjection, or the witch and the spirit medium. In *Beyond rationalism: Rethinking magic, witchcraft, and sorcery*, ed. Bruce Kapferer, 198–214. Berghahn Books.

Lang, P., and E. McAdam. 1995. Stories, giving accounts and systemic descriptions. *Human Systems* 6(2): 71–103.

Langness, L.L. 1967. Hysterical psychosis: The cross-cultural evidence. *American Journal of Psychiatry* 124(2): 143–152. doi:10.1176/ajp.124.2.143.

Lanius, Ruth A., Eric Vermetten, Richard J. Loewenstein, Bethany Brand, J. Christian Schmahl, Douglas Bremner, and David Spiegel. 2010. Emotion modulation in PTSD: Clinical and neurobiological evidence for a dissociative subtype. *American Journal of Psychiatry* 167(6): 640–647. doi:10.1176/appi.ajp.2009.09081168.

Lim, Young Mi, Isela Luna, Sandra L. Cromwell, Linda R. Phillips, Cynthia K. Russell, and Esperanza Torres de Ardon. 1996. Toward a cross-cultural understanding of family caregiving burden. *Western Journal of Nursing Research* 18(3): 252–66. doi:10.1177/019394599601800303.

Liotti, G. 2006. A model of dissociation based on attachment theory and research. *Journal of Trauma & Dissociation* 7(4): 55–73.

Liotti, Giovanni, and Andrew Gumley. 2008. An attachment perspective on schizophrenia: The role of disorganized attachment, dissociation and mentalization. In *Psychosis, trauma and dissociation: Emerging perspectives on severe psychopathology*, eds. Andrew Moskowitz, Ingo Schäfer, and Martin Justin Dorahy, 3769–4287. Chichester, West Sussex. UK: Wiley-Blackwell. Kindle file.

Littlewood, Roland. 1996. *Reason and necessity in the specification of the multiple self.* Royal Anthropological Institute.
Littlewood, Roland, and Maurice Lipsedge. 1987. The butterfly and the serpent: Culture, psychopathology and biomedicine. *Culture, Medicine and Psychiatry* 11(3): 289–335.
Lloyd, K.R., K.S. Jacob, V. Patel, L. St, D. Bhugra Louis, and A.H. Mann. 1998. The development of the short explanatory model interview (SEMI) and its use among primary-care attenders with common mental disorders. *Psychological Medicine* 28(05): 1231–1237.
Lopez, Kay A., and Danny G. Willis. 2004. Descriptive versus interpretive phenomenology: Their contributions to nursing knowledge. *Qualitative Health Research* 14(5): 726–735. doi:10.1177/1049732304263638.
Lucas, Richard. 2008. The psychotic wavelength. *Psychoanalytic Psychotherapy* 22(1): 54–63. doi:10.1080/02668730801962763.
Lucas, R.H., and R.J. Barrett. 1995. Interpreting culture and psychopathology: Primitivist themes in cross-cultural debate. *Culture, Medicine and Psychiatry* 19(3): 287–326.
Luhrmann, T.M., R. Padmavati, H. Tharoor, and A. Osei. 2015. Differences in voice-hearing experiences of people with psychosis in the USA, India and Ghana: Interview-based study. *The British Journal of Psychiatry* 206(1): 41–44. doi:10.1192/bjp.bp.113.139048.
Magana, Sandy M., Jorge I. Ramirez Garcia, Maria G. Hernandez, and Raymond Cortez. 2007. Psychological distress among latino family caregivers of adults with schizophrenia: The roles of burden and stigma. *Psychiatr Serv* 58(3): 378–84. doi:10.1176/appi.ps.58.3.378.
Maj, Mario. 2011. The rights of people with mental disorders: WPA perspective. *The Lancet* 378 (9802): 1534–1535. doi:10.1016/S0140-6736(11)60745-9.
Marneros, Andreas, and Frank Pillmann. 2004. *Acute and transient psychoses*. Cambridge: Cambridge University Press.
McLean, Duncan, Rangaswamy Thara, Sujit John, Robert Barrett, Peter Loa, John McGrath, and Bryan Mowry. 2014. DSM-IV "Criterion A" schizophrenia symptoms across ethnically different populations: Evidence for differing psychotic symptom content or structural organization? *Culture, Medicine and Psychiatry* 38(3): 408–426. doi:10.1007/s11013-014-9385-8.
McWilliam, Andrew. 2007. Austronesians in linguistic disguise: Fataluku cultural fusion in East Timor. *Journal of Southeast Asian Studies* 38(02): 355–375. doi:10.1017/S0022463407000082.
McWilliam, Andrew, and Elizabeth G. Traube. 2011a. Introduction. In *Land and life in Timor-Leste: Ethnographic essays*, eds. Andrew McWilliam, and Elizabeth G. Traube. Canberra, ACT, Australia: ANU E Press. EPUB file.
McWilliam, Andrew, and Elizabeth G. Traube (eds.). 2011b. *Land and life in Timor-Leste: Ethnographic essays*. Canberra, ACT, Australia: ANU E Press. EPUB file.
Mezzich, J.E., L.J. Kirmayer, A. Kleinman, H. Fabrega, D.L. Parron, B.J. Good, K.M. Lin, and S. M. Manson. 1999. The place of culture in DSM-IV. *The Journal of Nervous and Mental Disease* 187(8): 457–464.
Middleton, Hugh. 2015. *Psychiatry reconsidered: From medical treatment to supportive understanding*. Houndmills, Basingstoke, Hampshire; New York, NY: Palgrave Macmillan.
Miller, K.E., P. Omidian, A.S. Quraishy, N. Quraishy, M.N. Nasiry, S. Nasiry, N.M. Karyar, and A.A. Yaqubi. 2006. The Afghan symptom checklist: A culturally grounded approach to mental health assessment in a conflict zone. *American Journal of Orthopsychiatry* 76(4): 423–433.
Mitchell, Stephen A., and Lewis Ed Aron, eds. 1999. *Relational psychoanalysis: The emergence of a tradition* (Vol. 14). Relational Perspectives Book Series. Analytic Press. http://psycnet.apa.org/psycinfo/1999-02491-000.
Mizen, Richard. 2009. Some limitations of analysis. *Journal of Analytical Psychology* 54(4): 461–473. doi:10.1111/j.1468-5922.2009.01797.x.
Modvig, J., J. Pagaduan-Lopez, J. Rodenburg, C. Salud, R. Cabigon, and C. Panelo. 2000. Torture and trauma in post-conflict East Timor. *The Lancet* 356(9243): 1763
Mollica, R.F., Y. Caspi-Yavin, P. Bollini, T. Truong, S. Tor, and J. Lavelle. 1992. The Harvard trauma questionnaire. Validating a cross-cultural instrument for measuring torture, trauma, and

posttraumatic stress disorder in Indochinese refugees. *The Journal of Nervous and Mental Disease* 180(2): 111–116.
Morrison, Anthony P., Lucy Frame, and Warren Larkin. 2003. Relationships between trauma and psychosis: A review and integration. *British Journal of Clinical Psychology* 42(4): 331–353. doi:10.1348/014466503322528892.
Moskowitz, Andrew. 2008. Association and dissociation in the historical concept of schizophrenia. In *Psychosis, trauma and dissociation: Emerging perspectives on severe psychopathology*, eds. Andrew Moskowitz, Ingo Schäfer, and Martin Justin Dorahy, 1475–1903. Chichester, West Sussex. UK: Wiley-Blackwell. Kindle file.
Murphy, Dominic. 2008. Levels of explanation in psychiatry.' In *Philosophical issues in psychiatry: Explanation, phenomenology, and nosology*, eds. Kenneth S. Kendler, and Josef Parnas, 99–131. Johns Hopkins University Press.
Myers, Neely Laurenzo. 2010. Culture, stress and recovery from schizophrenia: Lessons from the field for global mental health. *Culture, Medicine and Psychiatry* 34(3): 500–528. doi:10.1007/s11013-010-9186-7.
Myers, Neely Laurenzo. 2011. Update: Schizophrenia across cultures. *Current Psychiatry Reports* 13(4): 305–311. doi:10.1007/s11920-011-0208-0.
Nijenhuis, Ellert R.S., and Onno van der Hart. 2011. Dissociation in trauma: A new definition and comparison with previous formulations. *Journal of Trauma & Dissociation* 12(4): 416–445. doi:10.1080/15299732.2011.570592.
Niner, Sarah. 2001. A long journey of resistance: The origins and struggle of CNRT. In *Bitter flowers, sweet flowers: East Timor, Indonesia, and the world community*, eds. Richard Tanter, Mark Selden, and Stephen Rosskamm Shalom, 15–29. Lanham, Maryland: Rowman & Littlefield.
Obeyesekere. 1984. *Medusa's hair: An essay on personal symbols and religious experience*. Chicago and London: University of Chicago Press. Kindle file.
Obeyesekere, Gananath. 1990. *The work of culture: Symbolic transformation in psychoanalysis and anthropology*. Chicago: University of Chicago Press.
Ortner, Sherry B. 2006. *Anthropology and social theory: Culture, power, and the acting subject*. Duke University Press.
Otto, Hiltrud, and Heidi Keller. 2014. *Different faces of attachment: Cultural variations on a universal human need.*
Patel, V., R. Araya, N. Chowdhary, M. King, B. Kirkwood, S. Nayak, G. Simon, and H.A. Weiss. 2008. Detecting common mental disorders in primary care in India: A comparison of five screening questionnaires. *Psychological Medicine* 38(02). doi:10.1017/S0033291707002334.
Patel, Vikram, and Shekhar Saxena. 2014. Transforming lives, enhancing communities—Innovations in global mental health. *New England Journal of Medicine* 370(6): 498–501. doi:10.1056/NEJMp1315214.
Pearce, W.Barnett. 2007. *Making social worlds: A communication perspective*. Oxford, UK: Blackwell.
Pillmann, F., A. Haring, S. Balzuweit, R. Blöink, and A. Marneros. 2000. Concordance of acute and transient psychoses and cycloid psychoses. *Psychopathology* 34(6):305–11.
Pillmann, Frank, Annette Haring, Sabine Balzuweit, Raffaela Blöink, and Andreas Marneros. 2003. Bouffée Délirante and ICD-10 acute and transient psychoses: A comparative study. *The Australian and New Zealand Journal of Psychiatry* 37(3): 327–333.
Read, U. 2012. I want the one that will heal me completely so it won't come back again: The limits of antipsychotic medication in rural Ghana. *Transcultural Psychiatry* 49(3–4): 438–460. doi:10.1177/1363461512447070.
Read, John, and Richard P. Bentall. 2012. Negative childhood experiences and mental health: Theoretical, clinical and primary prevention implications. *The British Journal of Psychiatry* 200(2): 89–91. doi:10.1192/bjp.bp.111.096727.
Read, J., B.D. Perry, A. Moskowitz, and J. Connolly. 2001. The contribution of early traumatic events to schizophrenia in some patients: A traumagenic neurodevelopmental model. *Psychiatry* 64(4): 319–345.

Read, J., J. Os, A.P. Morrison, and C.A. Ross. 2005. Childhood trauma, psychosis and schizophrenia: A literature review with theoretical and clinical implications. *Acta Psychiatrica Scandinavica* 112(5): 330–350.
Reis, R. 2013. Children enacting idioms of witchcraft and spirit possession as a response to trauma: Therapeutically beneficial, and for whom? *Transcultural Psychiatry* 50(5): 622–643. doi:10.1177/1363461513503880.
Renner, Walter, Ingrid Salem, and Klaus Ottomeyer. 2006. Cross-cultural validation of measures of traumatic symptoms in groups of asylum seekers from Chechnya, Afghanistan, and West Africa. *Social Behavior and Personality: An International Journal* 34(9): 1101–1114. doi:10.2224/sbp.2006.34.9.1101.
Renner, Walter, Ingrid Salem, and Klaus Ottomeyer. 2007. Posttraumatic stress in Asylum Seekers from Chechnya, Afghanistan, and West Africa: Differential findings obtained by quantitative and qualitative methods in three austrian samples. In *Cross-cultural assessment of psychological trauma and PTSD*, eds. John P. Wilson, and Catherine So-kum Tang. Inernational and Cultural Psychology. Springer.
Rodger, James. 2011. Beyond dualism and defamation: Utility and action. *The Psychiatrist* 35(11): 430–431. doi:10.1192/pb.35.11.430.
Rodger, James A. 2013. Avatar-assisted relational therapy for persecutory voices. *The British Journal of Psychiatry* 203(3): 233–234. doi:10.1192/bjp.203.3.233a.
Rodger, James, Sami Timimi, Joanna Moncrieff, Graham Behr, Carl Beuster, Pat Bracken, Ivor Browne, et al. 2014. Craddock and Mynors-Wallis's assault on thinking. *The British Journal of Psychiatry* 205(6): 497–498. doi:10.1192/bjp.205.6.497.
Rorty, Richard. 1989. *Contingency, irony, and solidarity*. Cambridge: Cambridge University Press.
Rosenfeld, Herbert. 2013. Contribution to the psychopathology of psychotic states. In *Projective identification: The fate of a concept*, 76, eds. Elizabeth Spillius, and Edna O'Shaughnessy. Routledge.
Ross, Colin A. 2006. *The trauma model: A solution to the problem of comorbidity in psychiatry*. Richardson, TX: Manitou Communications.
Ross, Colin A. 2008. Dissociative schizophrenia.' In *psychosis, trauma and dissociation: Emerging perspectives on severe psychopathology*, eds. Andrew Moskowitz, Ingo Schäfer, and Martin Justin Dorahy, 8433–8801. Chichester, West Sussex. UK: Wiley-Blackwell. Kindle file.
Saha, Sukanta, David Chant, Joy Welham, and John McGrath. 2005. A systematic review of the prevalence of schizophrenia. *PLoS Medicine* 2(5): e141. doi:10.1371/journal.pmed.0020141.
Sakti, Victoria Kumala. 2013. "Thinking too much": Tracing local patterns of emotional distress after mass violence in Timor-Leste. *The Asia Pacific Journal of Anthropology* 14(5): 438–454. doi:10.1080/14442213.2013.826733.
Scott, James, David Chant, Gavin Andrews, Graham Martin, and John McGRATH. 2007. Association between trauma exposure and delusional experiences in a large community-based sample. *The British Journal of Psychiatry* 190(4): 339–343. doi:10.1192/bjp.bp.106.026708.
Searles, Harold F. 1961. Phases of patient-therapist interaction in the psychotherapy of chronic schizophrenia. *The British Journal of Medical Psychology* 34: 169–193.
Seligman, Rebecca, and Laurence J. Kirmayer. 2008. Dissociative experience and cultural neuroscience: Narrative, metaphor and mechanism. *Culture, Medicine and Psychiatry* 32(1): 31–64.
Shevlin, Mark, James E. Houston, Martin J. Dorahy, and Gary Adamson. 2008. Cumulative traumas and psychosis: An analysis of the national comorbidity survey and the british psychiatric morbidity survey. *Schizophrenia Bulletin* 34(1): 193–199. doi:10.1093/schbul/sbm069.
Silove, Derrick. 2007. Adaptation, ecosocial safety signals, and the trajectory of PTSD. In *Understanding trauma: Integrating biological, clinical, and cultural perspectives*, eds. Laurence J. Kirmayer, Robert Lemelson, and Mark Barad, 242–258. Cambridge: Cambridge University Press.

Silove, Derrick, and Zachary Steel. 2006. Understanding community psychosocial needs after disasters: Implications for mental health services. *Journal of Postgraduate Medicine* 52(2): 121.

Silove, Derrick, and Philip B. Ward. 2014. Challenges in rolling out interventions for schizophrenia. *The Lancet*. doi:10.1016/S0140-6736(14)60085-4.

Silove, D., S. Ekblad, and R. Mollica. 2000. The rights of the severely mentally ill in post-conflict societies. *The Lancet* 355(9214): 1548–1549. doi:10.1016/S0140-6736(00)02177-2.

Silove, Derrick, Catherine Robina Bateman, Robert T. Brooks, C. Amaral Zulmira Fonseca, Zachary Steel, James Rodger, Ian Soosay, Greg Fox, Vikram Patel, and Adrian Bauman. 2008. Estimating clinically relevant mental disorders in a rural and an urban setting in postconflict Timor Leste. *Archives of General Psychiatry* 65(10): 1205–1212. doi:10.1001/archpsyc.65.10.1205.

Silove, Derrick, Robert Brooks, Catherine Robina Bateman Steel, Zachary Steel, Kalhari Hewage, James Rodger, and Ian Soosay. 2009. Explosive anger as a response to human rights violations in post-conflict Timor-Leste. *Social Science and Medicine* 69(5): 670–677. doi:10.1016/j.socscimed.2009.06.030.

Singh, Swaran P. 2011. Acute and transient psychotic disorders. In *Current themes in psychiatry in theory and practice*, eds. Niruj Agrawal, Jim Bolton, and Raghunandan Gaind, 77–98. London: Palgrave Macmillan.

Spiegel, David, Richard J. Loewenstein, Roberto Lewis-Fernández, Vedat Sar, Daphne Simeon, Eric Vermetten, Etzel Cardeña, and Paul F. Dell. 2011. Dissociative disorders in DSM-5. *Depression and anxiety* 28(9): 824–852. doi:10.1002/da.20874.

Steel, Zachary, Tien Chey, Derrick Silove, Claire Marnane, Richard A Bryant, and Mark van Ommeren. 2009. Association of torture and other potentially traumatic events with mental health outcomes among populations exposed to mass conflict and displacement: A systematic review and meta-analysis. *JAMA: The Journal of the American Medical Association* 302 (5):537–49. doi:10.1001/jama.2009.1132.

Stern, Daniel N. 2003. Introduction to the paperback edition. In *The interpersonal world of the infant: A view from psychoanalysis and developmental psychology*. Paperback Edition, xi–xxxix. London: Karnac Books.

Stevens, Janice. 1987. Brief psychoses: Do they contribute to the good prognosis and equal prevalence of schizophrenia in developing countries? *The British Journal of Psychiatry* 151(3): 393–396.

Sulaiman-Hill, Cheryl, and Sandra Thompson. 2010. Selecting instruments for assessing psychological wellbeing in afghan and kurdish refugee groups. *BMC Research Notes* 3(1): 237. doi:10.1186/1756-0500-3-237.

Summerfield, D. 2012. Afterword: Against "global mental health". *Transcultural Psychiatry* 49(3–4): 519–530. doi:10.1177/1363461512454701.

Taylor-Leech, Kerry. 2008. Language and identity in East Timor: The discourses of nation building. *Language Problems & Language Planning* 32(2): 153–180. doi:10.1075/lplp.32.1.04tay.

Taylor-Leech, Kerry. 2009. The language situation in Timor-Leste. *Current Issues in Language Planning* 10(1): 1–68.

Traube, Elizabeth G. 2007. Unpaid wages: Local narratives and the imagination of the nation. *The Asia Pacific Journal of Anthropology* 8(1): 9–25. doi:10.1080/14442210601161724.

Traube, Elizabeth G. 1986. *Cosmology and social life: Ritual exchange among the Mambai of East Timor*. Chicago: University of Chicago Press.

Traube, Elizabeth G. 2011. Painting the Flag. In *Land and life in Timor-Leste: Ethnographic essays*, eds. Andrew McWilliam, and Elizabeth G. Traube, 117–140. Canberra, ACT, Australia: ANU E Press. EPUB file

van der Hart, Onno, E. Witztum, and B. Friedman. 1993. From hysterical psychosis to reactive dissociative psychosis. *Journal of Traumatic Stress* 6(1): 43–64.

van der Hart, Onno, Ellert Nijenhuis, Kathy Steele, and Daniel Brown. 2004. Trauma-related dissociation: Conceptual clarity lost and found. *Australian and New Zealand Journal of Psychiatry* 38(11–12): 906–914. doi:10.1111/j.1440-1614.2004.01480.x.

van der Hart, Onno, and Eliezer Wiztum. 2008. Dissociative psychosis: Clinical and theoretical aspects. In *Psychosis, trauma and dissociation: Emerging perspectives on severe psychopathology*, eds. Andrew Moskowitz, Ingo Schäfer, and Martin Justin Dorahy, 7759–8118. Chichester, West Sussex. UK: Wiley-Blackwell. Kindle file.

van IJzendoorn, Marinus H., and Abraham Sagi-Schwartz. 2008. Cross-cultural patterns of attachment: Universal and contextual dimensions. In *Handbook of attachment*, eds. Jude Cassidy, and Phillip R. Shaver, 2nd ed., 880–905. New York, NY: Guilford Press.

Whitaker, Robert. 2010. Anatomy of an epidemic: Magic bullets, psychiatric drugs, and the astonishing rise of mental illness in America, 1st ed. Crown Publishing Group, Division of Random House Inc.

Wimmer, August. 2003. *Psychogenic psychoses* (Trans: Johan Schioldann). Adelaide, S. Aust.: Adelaide Academic Press. (Original work published 1916).

World Health Organisation (WHO). 1992. *The ICD-10 classification of mental and behavioural disorders: Clinical descriptions and diagnostic guidelines*. World Health Organisation.

Worsley, Peter. 1987. *Trumpet shall sound: A study of 'Cargo' cults in Melanesia*, 2nd ed. New York: Schocken.

Wunderink, L., R.M. Nieboer, D. Wiersma, S. Sytema, and F.J. Nienhuis. 2013. Recovery in remitted first-episode psychosis at 7 years of follow-up of an early dose reduction/discontinuation or maintenance treatment strategy: Long-term follow-up of a 2-year randomized clinical trial. *JAMA Psychiatry* 70(9): 913–920. doi:10.1001/jamapsychiatry.2013.19.

Yap, P.M. 1967. Classification of the culture-bound reactive syndromes. *Australian and New Zealand Journal of Psychiatry* 1(4): 172–179. doi:10.3109/00048676709159191.

Young, A. 1982. The anthropologies of illness and sickness. *Annual Review of Anthropology* 11 (1): 257–285.

Zarit, Steven H., Karen E. Reever, and Julie Bach-Peterson. 1980. Relatives of the impaired elderly: Correlates of feelings of burden. *The Gerontologist* 20(6): 649–655. doi:10.1093/geront/20.6.649.

Zatzick, Douglas F., Charles R. Marmar, Daniel S. Weiss, and Thomas Metzler. 1994. Does trauma-linked dissociation vary across ethnic groups? *The Journal of Nervous and Mental Disease* 182(10): 576–582.

Chapter 2
Traumatic Structural Dissociation and Its Cultural Dimensions

2.1 Why Dissociation?

Dissociation is a term used to describe a failure of integration of different psychic functions (mind-body; cognition-emotion; self-parts; mental functions etc.). There is debate as to whether the term should be used to describe normal experience, such as automatic driving and absorptive experiences, and whether pathological dissociation is qualitatively different from such normative dissociative-like states (Kirmayer 1994 and 2011; Nijenhuis and van der Hart 2011; van der Hart et al. 2004). The frequency and qualitative dimensions of dissociative experience also varies cross-culturally (Lewis-Fernández et al. 2007), as can be seen when comparing Western countries with non-Western settings where practice of trance and belief in spirit possession are more widespread. For anthropological purposes the use of term appears useful, since at a basic level it can be used initially for purely descriptive purposes, with theoretical models and assumptions put temporarily on hold. But as Seligman and Kirmayer (2008) note, when it comes to theorising, anthropological accounts of dissociative phenomena, while rich in attendance to context and social meaning, have remained disjointed from psychological and neurobiological understandings[1]; something which their own work seeks to partly address, and upon which we have built.

In this work we have drawn on specific models and contemporary research from multiple arenas, including cognitive and experimental psychology, psychoanalysis, neurobiology and anthropology, but hold that characterisations of dissociated states of mind are found both historically and cross-culturally (e.g. possession states), and have, in Rorty's (1989) words, been variously *redescribed* and represented in the

[1]Itself a further example of the epistemological tension between agentic and deterministic accounts of experience (see Sect. 1.7.2).

J. Rodger and Z. Steel, *Between Trauma and the Sacred*,
Cultural Studies of Science and Medicine, DOI 10.1007/978-3-319-24424-2_2

overlapping terminologies of many schools of Western psychology.[2] While acknowledging that the experience and concept of self-assumed within the Western psychological canon on dissociation may differ significantly from non-Western experience and constructs, the anthropological literature, including in relation to spirit-possession, can be read as supporting this broad definition of dissociation, with the proviso that lack of integration and externalised *experience* and attribution may be normative and not necessarily pathological (Seligman and Kirmayer 2008). Additionally important and efficacious cultural-work may *require* that such dissociated parts remain *unacknowledged* as *self*-parts (see Sects. 4.1.2—Footnote 2 and 5.2.1) and aspects of traumatic intrusions, might even be fruitfully understood, ontogenetically, as non-self (see Sects. 3.2 and 5.2.1—Footnote 14). Of course, the implicit theoretical assumptions, and subcultural understandings, embedded in different terminology, may itself shape both experience and outcome, through "social-looping" (see Sect. 1.7.2; Hacking 1999) and cultural scripting (see Sect. 5. 2.5). Nonetheless, whatever the various bottom-up and top-down forces involved, it is pertinent to note that dynamic brain imaging of changes in dissociable and discrete self-states supports their *subjective experiential* veracity (Littlewood 1996).

While the boundary between dissociative and everyday experience is obviously not always clearly defined, dissociative phenomena are accepted to be more common in non-Western settings. Certainly this was our experience in Timor-Leste where abrupt and apparently discontinuous changes in mental state, suggestive of dissociative shifts (albeit potentially culturally normative and adaptive ones) were commonly observed in many day-to-day encounters. These included culturally sanctioned contexts such as funerary and mourning rites (see Sect. 3.2), but also our research interviews (which sometimes appeared to precipitate a dissociative shift, unveiling previously masked distress, but sometimes facilitate a *sealing-over* of distress depending on the individual—see Sect. 1.4.3, Footnote 11). In both cultural and interview contexts, the abrupt shifts described were often precipitated by social cues although further cues later appeared to reconnect the individual with their earlier mental state, thereby restoring the continuity that appeared to have been lost.

Within the narrower research cohort of brief-remitting-relapsing (BRR) and acute-on-chronic (AOC) exacerbations of psychotic-like states under focus, and while not specific markers in themselves, there were also a number of features, suggestive of dissociative processes at work. These will be subsequently examined more extensively (see also Sect. 1.5) but in summary included:

1. Stereotyped descriptions/manifestations of psychotic symptoms with little variation between subjects. These included extreme states of agitation and aggression that appear to have rarely led to significant physical violence, suggesting such behaviour may have been partly "culturally scripted" (see Sect. 4.2.2).
2. Rapid onset in response to social stress or *symbolic triggers*, that sometimes included *dramatic* precursors or precipitants of onset and recurrence, such as

[2]Examples include a self "fragmented into a set of modules, subsystems, ego-states or part-selves, depending on the vocabulary chosen" (Ross 2008, Sect. 20.1.1).

episodes of collapse preceding an episode (see Sect. 2.3.4—Case BP5 and Table 2.1). While such precursors and triggers were often emotive, taken in isolation the subsequent response would appear unexpected and disproportionate. Resolution of symptoms was often equally rapid, often after a matter of hours or days, with occasional longer episodes.
3. Disavowal or genuine amnesia of disturbed behaviour (see Sect. 1.4.2—Table 1.3)
4. Some degree of *secondary gain*, in addition to the *primary gain* of temporarily sealing off distress from awareness, is often apparent to the impartial observer. This may include unsubtle gains such as exemption from certain family, social and occupational expectations, or more complex dynamics of *social redress* (see Sect. 4.2.2).
5. Disturbed behaviours were reported by families to respond to very small, doses of antipsychotic medication that may not be simply attributable to drug-naivety or racial pharmacogenomics (cf. Ninnemann 2012), but rather the "symbolic" power of Western medical treatment facilitating a sealing-over of distress (cf. van der Geest and Whyte 1989) although attitudes towards Western medicine and its interface with wider cultural dynamics are complex.[3]

We will also argue that there were many aspects of the psychosocial and cultural context at the time of our study in Timor-Leste that may have served to increase the likelihood of such dissociative phenomena. Dissociative states are often assumed to be *culturally pathoplastic* phenomena (Spiegel et al. 2011; see also Sect. 1.5), thereby explaining the fit between local factors and illness presentation, but once again how and why pathoplasticity come about is poorly understood and is an area we will attempt to conceptually develop. Finally dissociation may provide a useful model for at least *some psychotic states* (see Sect. 2.2.1), both being predicated on ideas of *failed psychic integration* (see Sect. 5.1). While there is burgeoning interest in this connection within the critical psychology field (e.g. Morrison et al. 2003; Moskowitz et al. 2008a, b) there are few modern studies that explore this link in non-Western settings. Guinness's (1992) and Castillo's (1994) work are notable exceptions but remain in need of updating.

The dissociative formulation outlined in this work commences with an exploration of trauma-informed linear models of dissociative phenomena, and how they can contribute to an explanation of psychotic or psychotic-like mental states and behaviour, but further considers how traumatic events may become symbolically encoded and re-triggered, in the context of Timorese practice and belief. We will also go onto consider how unconscious motivation, conflict and phantasy, further shape dissociative-psychotic responses (Chap. 3) and how the recursive interaction of cultural factors further interact with this process (Chap. 4)—factors arguably critical to the unique patterns of dissociative phenomena in different parts of the world.

[3]Several individuals and families articulated a degree of faith in Western medicine, although there was also disappointment (see Sect. 5.2.4) and ambivalence and such faith is moving in the opposing direction to forces promoting cultural revitalisation (Sect. 4.2.3). We also need to be aware of how our positioning as doctors may have influenced responses (Csordas et al. 2010; Sect. 1.7.1).

2.2 The Model of Traumatic (Structural) Dissociation

The clearest *linear model* of dissociative experience is the trauma model. Also known as the model of structural dissociation, it designates dissociative states as pathological, albeit perhaps understandable and even partially adaptive, responses to trauma (van der Hart et al. 2004). Rehabilitating and refining the observations and theorising of Pierre Janet,[4] trauma theorists, van der Hart et al. (2004) have argued that a breakdown of integration between different parts of the psyche, on account of predisposing vulnerability and later trauma induced cognitive and affective overload, to result in the splitting or fragmentation of self-experience, into psychobiological subsystems, along pre-existing fault lines dictated by evolutionary psychobiology. For example, in elaborating on Myers' observations from World War I, they argue a split might emerge, along the most basic fault lines, between subsystems underpinning *rational-thought* and *feeling*; or between *approach* and *retreat* (van der Hart et al. 2004).[5] Additional trauma may then further fragment these defensive or goal-directed self-subsystems; for example defensive subsystems may become further divided to include *freeze*, *flight* and *hypervigilance* (van der Hart et al. 2004).

While some aspects of semantic, episodic and procedural memory may be shared by different self-subsystems, others may become tied to a specific domain of the psyche (Castillo 1994)—particularly highly emotive, traumatic events that become encoded when the field of consciousness is adaptively narrowed to deal with the threatening event or injury, which lacking wider contextual links requires the recreation of the same intense emotional state, or specific triggers to *activate* them (cf. Kirmayer 1994 on state-dependent learning). Poor recall *across* different parts of self would therefore be predicted. Amnesia, following the brief-psychotic states described, might be expected, if they are indeed dissociative in origin, as such experience would be rapidly *walled-off* following the removal of key triggers.

However implicit in the model of structural dissociation model is the recognition that dissociative responses are imperfect in sealing-over distress, and become problematic for the individual, and those close to them, even when "successful" (Seligman and Kirmayer 2008; van der Hart et al. 2004). *Positive* and painful dissociative phenomena may emerge when embodied experiences and memories from one self-subsystem intrude into consciousness, yet, when successfully sealed-over, a sense of deficit or loss may be *felt* or apparent to others, due to the removal of significant self-experience and affective range from the dominant

[4]Janet (1869–1947) is described as the French founding father of the "new dynamic psychiatry" before Freud (Ellenberger 1981).

[5]Van der Hart et al. (2004, 907), following Myers, have divided the healthy and traumatised parts of the self into the "apparently normal part of the personality" and "the emotional part of the personality" respectively, although we have not followed this cultural convention here.

self-domain (van der Hart et al. 2004).[6] Greater difficulties in effectively walling-off experience may also become apparent as the initial narrow range of trigger stimuli become widened due to the subsequent pairing of conditionally emergent, imperfectly sealed, affective experiences with new contexts, thereby providing the material for new conditioned cues (van der Hart et al. 2004).

2.2.1 Traumatic Dissociation: From PTSD to Psychosis

A range of PTSD symptoms—not limited to the ones thought of as classically dissociative—can then be conceptualised via this model. As such *positive*, or intrusive, dissociative experiences may entail *psychoform-phenomena* from both the *re-experiencing* (intrusive thoughts, flashbacks, nightmares, emotional reliving) and *hyperarousal* (anger, hypervigilance, hyperstartle) dimensions of PTSD[7] (van der Hart et al. 2004). The more commonly understood dissociative symptoms of PTSD (complete or partial amnesia, and a sense of detachment) then become understandable as the *negative* (or deficit) correlates of these positive dissociative phenomena, that can be expanded to include other symptoms, such as *restricted range of affect* (van der Hart et al. 2004).

In clinical contexts, traumatised individuals may have a predominantly *intrusive-hypervigilant*, or a predominantly *emotional overmodulation-numbing* clustering of symptoms (Lanius et al. 2010). While peritraumatic dissociation has been shown to be a significant risk-factor for the development of PTSD symptoms, it seems likely that it may also give rise to a symptom profile more dominated by emotional numbing and less objective physiological arousal (Griffin et al. 1997) as the initial traumatic experience remains at least partially sealed-off, except when triggered or brought to the fore by other factors. In contrast the absence of peritraumatic dissociation, might be predicted to lead to a PTSD profile more dominated by re-experiencing and hyperarousal symptoms (cf. Lanius et al. 2010). This model also predicts *fluctuation* between intrusive dissociative experience and deficit states, in response to changes in the perceived level of stress or threat, in addition to other factors (see Sect. 5.3—Fig. 5.1), and such fluctuation between "intrusions into and withdrawals from the executive self" has been well described in clinical work with dissociative conditions (Ross 2008, Sect. 1.4; cf. Lanius et al. 2010) and indeed are described by Ross (2008, Sect. 1.3) as "the predominant cause of a symptoms in a structurally dissociated psyche."

---

[6]Relational psychoanalysts may speak of sensing the missing emotion in the counter-transference (Wallin 2007).

[7]Most factor analytic studies exploring PTSD symptom-clusters have confirmed the basis for separating out *re-experiencing*, *hyperarousal* and *avoidance* symptom dimensions, but have also pointed to the need to separate out a further dimension of emotional numbing (Pietrzak and Southwick 2009).

Additionally it is now understood that dissociative experiences can include *somatoform phenomena* (van der Hart et al. 2000). Intrusive somatoform phenomena may include pain or other somatic sensations, that may represent unprocessed and poorly integrated embodied memories of painful experience, or even ongoing physiological pain, split off, or repressed, from active awareness (van der Hart et al. 2000). Negative correlates of somatoform symptoms would then include, experiences of non-organic sensory loss (including blindness or deafness) and paralysis (van der Hart et al. 2000) and need not resort to "symbolic" Freudian explanations of intrapsychic conflict and conversion (although need not be mutually exclusive of such explanations—see Sect. 3.1.4).

In this light, the difference between flashbacks and hallucinations may not be as clear as descriptive psychopathologists would like. Rather flashbacks might be defined as intrusive perceptual phenomena in which the insight and awareness that one is re-experiencing events from the past is at least partially retained, or only very briefly lost. In some instances, "hallucinations" may then represent perceptually and aetiologically similar processes but in which this awareness or memory of the begetting trauma is lost (Read et al. 2005). For example due to the narrowing of attention, or peritraumatic dissociation, affecting encoding during the traumatic experience; different sensory aspects of the traumatic memory may be subsequently recalled in a piecemeal manner, or may be fully recalled but lack the contextual mnemenic embedding that allow their identification with the past, rather than the present (Read et al. 2005). Additionally "hallucinations" might also represent *variations* on a traumatic-theme, or *symbolic*-representations, of earlier trauma (Hardy et al. 2005), further complicating awareness and insight into their origin.

Since trauma is often re-lived in multiple sensory modalities, the proposed shared ontogenetic basis of "flashbacks" and certain hallucinatory experiences, may provide an alternative explanation as to why visual and tactile "hallucinations" (conventionally often seen as a marker of organic brain disturbance) are not uncommonly represented, alongside more traditional "auditory hallucinations," in psychotic symptomatology partly attributed to trauma, and was consistent with our own recording of such symptoms in the BRR group (see Sect. 1.4.2—Table 1.3).

Similarly *hypervigilance* secondary to traumatic experience may become generalised and de-contextualised, manifesting as paranoid ideation, or misattributed and misdirected leading to the development of more specific persecutory delusions (Moskowitz et al. 2009; Read et al. 2005). If hallucinations are sometimes a form of de-contextualised flashback, the inaccessibility to memory of the historical cause may then trigger a different set of secondary attributions that appear delusional. Additionally any associated de-contextualised emotional experiences may further contribute to misattribution or be associated with a particular phenomenology such as the genesis of "delusional atmosphere" (Moskowitz et al. 2008a, b; Read et al. 2005).

Several researchers have also commented on the similarity between the so called *negative symptoms* of schizophrenia and the cognitive and emotional deficits seen in chronic and/or dissociative subtypes of PTSD (Morrison et al. 2003; Read et al. 2005; Stampfer 1990) in which charged-emotional states may be largely sealed-off.

The intrusion–withdrawal model, also provides a basis for considering *passivity phenomena* such as thought insertion/withdrawal and "made emotions" or "made actions" that are included amongst so called First Rank Symptoms (FRS) of schizophrenia (Ross 2008).

It is important to note that, following Ross (2008, Sect. 20.1), we also view the model of psychotic-dissociation described here as "entirely consistent with the structural model of dissociation" but advocate an extension and broadening of its logical implications. We acknowledge with Ross that this goes beyond what is intended by the pioneers of this model who continue to assert that the concept of dissociation should be limited to instances involving a "division of an individual's personality" such that each "dissociative part of the personality, minimally includes its own at least rudimentary first-person perspective" (Nijenhuis and van der Hart 2011, 418). In response Ross (2014, 285) rightly raises this as a threshold question, and asks "how rudimentary can…personality…be and still qualify as structural dissociation?" More specifically in the context of dissociative model of psychosis he quotes Bleuler's assertion, from his seminal *Dementia Praecox or the Group of Schizophrenias* (Ross 2008, Sect. 20.0) that "even emotionally charged ideas or drives attain a degree of autonomy so that the personality falls to pieces" suggesting the possibility of dissociative fragments of the psyche, at a much more rudimentary level than that captured by the concept of personality is possible (see also Sect. 3.2). As such this is consistent with theories and observations of both personality preservation (Johannessen et al. 2007) and "personality disintegration" (Chung 2007, 2) in persons diagnosed with psychosis and may reflect the success or otherwise respectively of sealing-over intrusive symptom. Preservation of the personality has been particularly noted in brief-psychotic states (McCabe and Strömgren 1975) and in Chaps. 4 and 5 (for summary diagram see Sect. 5.3—Fig. 5.1) we will explore an array of sociocultural processes that may mitigate against disintegrative forces, fostering a degree of integration, or at least psychic-organisation. Where genuine integration occurs, *constructive* and lasting personality change would be predicted.

Evidence for the Trauma-Psychosis Model

In recent years there has been a convergence of evidence linking trauma, both in childhood and as an adult, to an increased risk of psychosis. This holds both at a general level but also to specific symptoms. Studies have now moved well beyond evidence of simple association, and can be argued to provide strong corroboration of causal models according to Bradford Hill's (1965) well-established criteria of strength and consistency of association, dose-response gradient (through stratification of trauma exposure) and directionality (through prospective studies) (for comprehensive reviews see Morrison et al. 2003; Read et al. 2005, 2008). These obviously need to be considered alongside the interrelated criteria of psycho-biological plausibility, analogy, and scientific coherence, which we have partly addressed above, and will return to in the final chapter (see Sect. 5.1).

Studies using dose-response stratification of trauma-exposure are also illustrative for our purposes, and while mainly conducted in high-income, industrial Western countries, also highlight the impact of cumulative trauma and adversity, characteristic of the population studied in Timor-Leste.[8] For example, large scale epidemiological studies quantifying retrospective-trauma exposure and using validated structured diagnostic interviews, in the United States measuring *childhood* trauma, and in the United Kingdom measuring trauma in *adult* life, generated an adjusted psychosis-prediction odds-ratio (OR) of 7.4 and 18 respectively for those who had experienced 3 different trauma-types, and an exponential increase to an OR of 30.2 and 193 respectively, for those who had experienced the maximum of 5 trauma-types[9] (Shevlin et al. 2008). A smaller scale, but well-designed study in the Netherlands (Janssen et al. 2004, 41), also retrospectively stratified trauma-exposure and severity in childhood, but prospectively explored development of psychotic illness using a structured diagnostic interview, and similarly reported that:

> subjects who reported abuse in the highest frequency category had an estimated 30 times greater chance to develop a needs-based diagnosis of psychosis compared to those not exposed to childhood abuse. Less frequent abuse was associated with an estimated five times greater risk to develop a need-based diagnosis of psychosis compared to those without any exposure to childhood abuse.

In examining the impact on individual symptoms, the evidence is strongest for positive-symptoms, in particular for hallucinations, but less consistent for delusions.[10] However again in larger studies and those stratifying levels of cumulative trauma and adversity, dose-response and arguably causal associations are also found for paranoid ideation (Bentall et al. 2012) and delusions (Scott et al. 2007), comparable with risk levels for hallucinations. For example, Bentall et al. (2012)

---

[8]Supporting our explanation of traumatic origins it appears noteworthy that the average lifetime experience of traumatic event in the BRR psychotic cohort in Timor-Leste were higher (mean 7.8, s.d. 3.1) than the screened population as a whole (mean 4.2, s.d., 2.6) although lower than those who were identified with a diagnosis of PTSD (mean 15.3, s.d. 6.4). This latter finding however is unsurprising given that by definition those with simple PTSD are likely to be ruminating about traumatic experiences and experiencing intrusive recollections of such experiences, whereas (according to our argument) BRR psychotic symptoms may *seal-over* day-to-day memories and acknowledgement of trauma and associated emotional distress, through a culturally shaped dissociative process, potentially affecting questionnaire responses relating to such events.

[9]Although we might expect greater psychosis-risk to be associated with childhood trauma, a higher risk in this analysis was associated with the British study measuring trauma in *adult* life (Shevlin et al. 2008). However this latter British study did not concurrently measure predisposing childhood-trauma in victimised adults and since childhood trauma predisposes to later adult victimisation (Widom et al. 2008), an association that holds in suffers of psychosis (Bebbington et al. 2011), it seems likely that the study of adult trauma would have concurrently subsumed many histories of childhood trauma. This is consistent with epidemiological risk models of psychosis, which report high rates of both childhood and adult trauma in psychotic persons (P.E. Bebbington et al. 2004).

[10]However, since delusions are often modelled as arising from misinterpretations of anomalous experience such as hallucinations, and such models predict that not all those who experience hallucinations will develop a delusional explanation, it is not surprising that the association between trauma and delusions is slightly less robust than for hallucinations (according to Bradford-Hill's consistency-replicability across studies).

measured and stratified retrospectively recalled childhood-trauma against paranoid-ideation and voice-hearing experiences quantified by the Psychosis Screening Questionnaire. While a single reported childhood adverse event was associated with an adjusted OR of paranoid ideation and auditory- hallucinations of 3.3 and 2.3 respectively, risk increased exponentially to 17.5 and 14.8 respectively, in the presence of 4 or more reported adversities. A similar recent study (Muenzenmaier et al. 2015) measuring and stratifying both retrospective trauma alongside aspects of the wider family environment (which may be protective or lack protective influence perhaps partly analogous with a conflict-torn environment like Timor-Leste) and utilising structured diagnostic interviews in place of screening tools, found a similar, although more modest, dose-response ratio for both delusional experiences and hallucinations.

In further support and illustration of our hypothesis a large-scale Australian study (Scott et al. 2007) retrospectively stratifying trauma-exposure and using structured diagnostic interviews, found evidence of delusional experiences associated with trauma, could be in the presence or absence of concurrent symptoms of PTSD (the latter perhaps representing a state of more effective *sealing-over* of intrusive trauma symptoms; see also Sect. 1.6, Footnote 22). Particularly relevant to our own work in Timor-Leste, some of the strongest predictors of concurrent delusions (all with a relative-risk (RR) > 7) included: being physically attacked, threatened with a weapon or tortured; involvement in combat; or witnessing someone close to you harmed or killed. Again an exponential increase in risk of endorsement of delusional experience was documented from a RR of 2.5 in those reporting 1–2 trauma types, to 9.5 in those reporting 5 or more trauma-types.

There is less direct evidence of an association with trauma in *negative-symptoms* of psychosis, although such subjects may be difficult to recruit in sufficient numbers as lack of volition and motivation may represent important aspects of the clinical picture. Additionally negative-symptoms often develop later in the disorder's trajectory, often in the context of multiple relapses, in which case the recollection of trauma may be more tenuous, confounded with the trauma of recurrent admissions and a subsuming illness-narrative. Finally presentations dominated by negative symptoms, may represent a deficit-dissociative state, in which active memories and emotions of trauma are dissociative sealed-off, or defended against, and therefore not available for recall.

Finally there is little research looking into associations between trauma and *passivity phenomena*, except to note that studies have in fact found higher rates of first-rank symptoms (FRS) in dissociative identity disorder (DID), with its more explicit traumatic aetiology, than in schizophrenia[11] (Laddis and Dell 2012; Ross et al. 1990). These were not elicited in our subjects, but would have required subject openness and recall, alongside translator linguistic dexterity, so neither could we

[11]For schizophrenia such FRS were once considered pathognomonic and retain some diagnostic weighting in DSM-IV-TR and ICD-10 (although have been downgraded in significance with the publication of DSM-5; APA 2013, 810).

confidently say that they were absent (for discussion on the cultural dimension on such phenomena however see Sect. 5.2.1).

We will return to a review of neuropsychological evidence linking trauma, dissociation and psychosis (see Sect. 5.1) in which we also go on to consider the relationship between brief and chronic psychosis (see Sect. 5.2).

2.3 Trauma and Symbol

2.3.1 *Trauma Can Arise from Bodily and/or Symbolic Threat or Injury*

Whereas conventionally trauma is defined as arising from events involving actual threat to bodily integrity (of self or others), "symbolic trauma" might be defined as involving threats to the integrity of important individual and communal beliefs and systems of meaning, critical to the individual's and group's concepts of life and selfhood. Both types of trauma are of course intensely real to the sufferers and may commonly co-exist, or represent overlapping dimensions of a single act/violation—as in military rape (Littlewood 1997).

A particularly well documented example of symbolic trauma (although undisputedly co-existing with gross bodily and material human rights violations) is that experienced by Tibetan citizens and refugees resulting from the systematic destruction and confiscation of public and private Tibetan Buddhist symbols (including temples, monasteries and monuments, together with private texts, flags, prayer wheels and photos), alongside the total prohibition of the outward expression of Tibetan Buddhist practices and sentiments, through which their cultural identity and sense of self was articulated and constituted (Janes 1995). While a study investigating the cross-cultural applicability and relevance of Western concepts of traumatic-experience concluded that such concepts were meaningful for Tibetan refugees exiled in India, and who were believed to have undergone only minimal Western acculturation, the researchers identified a critical need, for this group, to expand notions of traumatic experience to include the impact of the kind of symbolic traumas described above (Terheggen et al. 2001). Indeed when eleven independent Tibetan assessors were asked to rank traumatic experience according to likely impact and distress, "destruction of religious signs", "leaving home for political reasons", and "being forbidden to live according to one's own religion" were consistently rated first, second and third, ahead of "feeling one's life is in danger" which was ranked forth (Terheggen et al. 2001, 397).

Despite little take-up of Christian Catholicism during the period of Portuguese administration, the majority of East-Timorese subsequently overwhelmingly identified with, and converted to, the Roman Catholic church, which had become a symbol and bastion of the resistance movement, and a public thorn in the side of the Indonesian regime (Kohen 2001) notwithstanding very visible attempts at appeasement of the church by Indonesian authorities.[12] During the independence struggle the attempted incrimination of Catholic leaders, including the iconic resistance leader Bishop Belo, and the desecration of religious buildings, for example through their appropriation into houses of torture, might be seen as another aspect of symbolic trauma (Aditjondro 2000), not dissimilar to the religious oppression described in Tibet. Traube (2007) further describes the extensive destruction of traditionally sacred sites (mythically enshrined "origin villages") by pro-independence militia, in her work with Mambai people in the mountainous district of Aileu, 40 kilometres south of the Dili.

In Timor, the killing or loss of animals was also described by the ex-patriate service director of Timor's fledgling mental health service, *Saude Mental*, as eliciting a greater and more protracted degree of distress than might be expected from their loss of their material value alone (pers. comm.). Perhaps because, as observed by Hicks (2004) in his ethnography of the Tetum in the 1970s, certain animals—in particular buffalo, but also pigs—are associated with a high degree of social prestige, and form key components of important ritual transactions such as bridal wealth and ritual sacrifices (where the spilling of animal blood provides an important conduit between the living and ancestral dead). The spilling of animal blood by the enemy appears then as an affront and aberration of this symbolism. This was particularly perversely illustrated by the case of a young woman we interviewed from the wider non-psychotic cohort, meeting ongoing criteria for severe PTSD. *She described witnessing a wide range of atrocities, including the slaughter and consumption of 20 family pigs and goat. Furthermore she reported she herself was then made to drink the blood of the animals which militia had dipped with the Indonesian flag.*

The understanding of symbolic trauma we have developed here overlaps with what Litz et al. (2009) have termed "moral injury." They define this as "not merely a state of cognitive dissonance, but a state of loss of trust in previously deeply held beliefs about one's own or others' ability to keep our shared moral covenant" (Nash and Litz 2013, 368). Sakti's (2013, 441) ethnographic fieldwork in the Western Baiqueno speaking enclave of Oecussi illustrated just such a broken covenant—alongside broken kinship networks of exchange and ritual obligation earlier described (Sect. 1.6)—when interviewing a father whose son had been killed by local Indonesian sponsored militia in a brutal post-Independence ballot massacre, the father lamented: "'Our *brothers* from our *brothering* village took our *children* and *fathers* away from us'" [italics in original].

[12]This included the erection, at considerable expense and technical difficulty, of an enormous, 27 meter high, effigy of Christ the King (Portuguese Cristo Rei), high on a hilltop overlooking Dili's harbour (similar to that overlooking Lisbon, and the Cristo Redentor, overlooking Rio de Janeiro,). Unveiled by Indonesian President Suharto himself in 1996, the statue was envisioned as a gift to the Timorese people, to commemorate twenty years of Indonesian "integration" (Aditjondro 2000).

As with symbolic trauma, it clearly co-exists alongside physical trauma and threat to life, and appears to be associated with intrusive symptoms,[13] including *traumatic re-experiencing* (Litz et al. 2009) that based on the model developed here might include hallucinatory-like content.

2.3.2 Belief Itself Can Be Traumatic

In cultures, where threats from unseen but presumed potent "symbolic realities" are ever present, one can argue for causation of mental illness, and perhaps even death, from simply the belief alone that one has become a victim of sorcery (or of allied sources of harm; Hahn and Kleinman 1983). Anthropological studies have convincingly demonstrated a link between such imprecations, accusations, counter-measures, and the community's response; and the wider psychosocial dynamics of material inequality, jealousy, trauma and loss common to all societies (Evans-Pritchard 1976; Niehaus et al. 2001) which was a view supported by aspersions of sorcery in our study. In all we interviewed eight persons in which sorcery/witchcraft was mentioned, predominantly as culturally validated cause of misfortune or distress, and sometimes but not necessarily crossing severity thresholds associated with mental health diagnosis. Significantly sorcery was not described as a cause of psychosis except in one person who cited it half-heartedly, amongst a number of other possible causes (see Sect. 2.3.3—Case BP3 below). Although in one interview the subject identified his mother as a witch, accused of harming others (but not the son himself), this was arguably a symptom of psychosis not shared or validated by other family or community members (but nonetheless with implications reflecting a shared cultural logic; see Sect. 2.3.4—Case BP4). In two persons fear of sorcery was reinforced by the transmogrified appearance of a sorcerer in dreams (which relates to the night-time when they are thought to attack their victims while asleep—again see Sect. 2.3.4).

Accusations were not directed at specific others in our presence which may have been because direct aspersions of such would have serious implications for both victim and the accused in accordance with traditional systems of justice.[14] Notions of witchcraft and sorcery may however be tacitly subsumed in wider beliefs in

[13]Whether symbolic trauma or moral injury on its own would lead to intrusive rather than simply ruminative experience is unclear—studies of moral injury, generally involving military veterans, generally include trauma that has a concurrent dimension of physical threat, injury or loss (whether as victim or perpetrator). The model predicts that where physical and moral injuries co-occur, symptoms and/or impairment will be more severe. As we shall go onto explore (see Chap. 4) it may be that the loss of containing meaning rendered by moral injury, leads to an uncoupling of the memory and affect associated with physical trauma, now untethered and subject to recurrent intrusion into daily experience.

[14]For example amongst the Tetum-speaking community, described by Hicks (2004, 88) in the eastern district of Viqueque, *historically* "death was the traditional punishment for … sorcery" and no doubt required "proof" with consequences for false-allegations.

particular the *fulan lotuk* (see Sect. 2.3.4) or projected onto *rai nain* rather than the human world. Beyond sorcery, the belief in unseen spirits appeared widespread—throughout different strata of society and across different parts of the country, including the capital—and has formed an important focus of much historical and contemporary ethnography (e.g. Bovensiepen 2011; Hicks 2004). Once distressing experiences have been attributed to a specific cultural cause, such as *rai nain* or the *fulan lotuk*, by the individual and those around him/her, the meaning and implicit cultural prognosis may create a social-looping process confirming the individuals fate (see Sect. 1.7.2; Seligman and Kirmayer 2008; cf. Hacking 1999), or necessitating counter-measures which if followed may bring about recovery (Kapferer 1979).

Case BP2

Such was the case with Ricardo, a 60 year old man, who believed, with his wife, that he was under the spell of the "fulan lotuk." Back in his late thirties for three years he had experienced intermittent visual hallucinations. This first began when he was on his way home late one evening and, having lost his way, entered a coconut farm. When he left the farm he felt drunk, despite having consumed no alcohol, and he felt the place he was in was very different from the material world. He heard a rustling sound and states he then saw a large fluctuating white and red non-human creature as "big as a house". It followed him home although he states he was not scared—as although he did not know what it was, he thought it might have been from God and he knew it not to be evil. Subsequently it would appear to him about once or twice a week when he was walking, including when his family was present, although they could not see it. He thinks it may have occurred because he did something wrong while walking through the coconut farm, and he didn't say sorry. He recalled that five small rocks were thrown to him at this time. He kept them and for two years he acted as a healer (killing chickens and divining by looking at their hearts). He would tell people whether they would die, or the cause of their pregnancy loss (such as jealousy by other people). He also performed some ceremonies for spirits. After two years, another healer took the stones, telling him that they would make him crazy and he has not been a healer since.

The stones "found" by Ricardo and their linkage to his encounter with the non-human entity have a strong resonance to Hicks' (2004) description of men encountering stones believed to harbour *rai nain*, powerful nature spirits, who subsequently appear to the finder in dreams in order to establish a relationship and covenant with it. *Rai nain* were described by Hicks' informants of being capable of bestowing significant power of the finder, but also great misfortune, including illness and death, should the covenant be broken, and Hicks describes an elaborate ritual protocol to be followed in such situations. Although Ricardo was still affected by the *fulan lotuk* his current symptoms consisted mainly of feeling a "bit drunk", sleeping an hour or two less a night, and being angry and argumentative with his wife and grown-up children for two to three days each month, during which he often takes himself off into the fields. Although there may be links with trauma (see Table 2.1), his age, gender and social position, and wider local and national context; *at the level of belief* it may be that the healers actions in removing the stones had delimited the spirits influence in the mutually influencing eyes of Ricardo, his family and surrounding community, and mitigating any potentially malignant social looping process. According to one cultural consultant, it is recognised that people who have recovered from a state of *bulak* may still be influenced by the *fulan lotuk* but in a less dramatic manner, consistent with Ricardo's story.

2.3.3 Trauma Can Be Encoded Symbolically

That is to say that an individual's experience or witnessing of physical threat, injury or loss may be ascribed symbolic significance and processed in these terms. Salient personal and cultural meanings may therefore be closely linked to the actual events influencing how such events are encoded and subsequently recalled, retrieved or involuntary elicited from memory stores. For example in Timor-Leste, illness or misfortune might be interpreted in terms of violation of sacred (*lulik*) codes, or taboos in relation to the ancestors or local spirits (*rai-nain*). Even where death was ascribed as secondary to natural causes, or as the result of armed conflict, as both Hicks (2004) and Traube (1986) confirm, the passage of the deceased person's soul to the secure and desired realm of the ancestors is fraught with danger. Deviations from proscribed ritual practices, participated in at fixed points for a fixed period following a death, and designed to ensure the smooth transition of the deceased's soul to the ancestral realm—alongside death believed to have occurred in the first place due to *lulik* violations—may therefore leave the soul in an indeterminate and unhappy state, free to "haunt" remaining kin in the land of the living to remind them of their dereliction of duty (Hicks 2004). Such beliefs and practices remained evident in present day Timor-Leste, across social strata.

Case BP3
The relevance of this was clearly illustrated by Dores, a 24 year old who was tormented by recurrent and distressing visual and tactile hallucinations, of soldiers in uniform coming into her room every night, sometimes touching her. In response she would often shout, indicating a desire to be left alone ("get away from me" or "I don't want to go with you, go home its cold"), but sometimes responses that were harder to make sense of (for example, "its raining, I am going to climb the mountain with many people"). She also claimed to see the spirits of the dead, including her own grandparents.

Dores lived in one of a cluster of small building occupied by extended kin and other families. Family members and co-residents described her as "bulak" and her distress was also stated to be worse during the "fulan lotuk." While she had initially endorsed the items of "involvement in a combat situation during Indonesian times" and having "witnessed the murder of strangers around the time of the 1999 vote" on the HTQ, on later interview she denied experiencing significant trauma, and her family appeared sceptical, although she indicated a desire talk in private "to give us the whole story." What was clear was that her own father had been killed in 1984 by the Indonesian military, when she was still very young.

While there were some features of her presentation that suggest a possible organic contribution, including previous malaria in the year it began, alongside drowsiness and somatic symptoms that predictably prefigured her nightly "hallucinatory" symptoms; her fevers had long since resolved, and she had apparently seen medical practitioners on three occasions with no physical cause for her experiences identified (although procedures such as EEG and brain imaging were not available in this setting). There were potential complex social and family tensions that may be relevant to understanding her symptoms, and she was unusual in being treated with little sympathy, sometimes even mockingly, by some family members and co-residents. Outside of home however she appeared to show a relatively high level of functioning and social adjustment. She was actively pursuing higher education, which she reported enjoying although feeling stressed by, but reported she was coping with the workload, and had many friends.

As well as doctors, she had seen a traditional healer on several occasions about her symptoms. While various explanations were offered by Dores and family members, Dores appeared to accept (at least publically) the idea that she had this problem primarily because Indonesian soldiers killed her father but his body was not properly buried. The healers needed to perform another rite to appease the spirit of her dead father, having apparently done this once before, after which she said she had improved a little.

2.3.4 The Symbol Itself May Be Sufficient to Trigger Distress

Symbols through which memories of trauma and loss have become encoded and entwined, may themselves be sufficient to evoke involuntary recollection of these events, together with their associated meanings and emotions. Such symbols may be identical to those implicated in encoding (see Table 2.1—trauma and *lulik* factors), or related through association. They may be configured in time, or in place, or both. The clearest example of such a temporally configured symbol in the current cohort is the reoccurring periodicity of the *fulan lotuk*, which was the most common trigger of brief-psychotic recurrence or exacerbation (in 7/10 of the BRR cohort and 4/4 of the AOC cohort respectively). It was unclear whether, and under what conditions, the *fulan lotuk* was considered causal in relation to *initial* presentations of mental distress; although on direct probing it was sometimes ambivalently cited as such. It appeared however to represent a common *aggravator of pre-existing vulnerabilities* associated with other *lulik* factors, perhaps linked by principles of association (see Sect. 3.1.2).

Other important symbols configured in both time and space included both public and private *lulik* rituals and ceremonies. A commanding example of a significant public ceremony was the *mate bien* (lit. good death). This was a traditional public festival celebrating the ancestors that in Catholic times had become amalgamated with All Soul's Day. In more recent years it had become a contemporary memorial day to those who lost their lives in the Independence struggle. The most important private ceremonies also pertained to the deceased and involved a series of ritual celebrations at prescribed times over a fixed period (the duration and frequency of which may vary according to ethnolinguistic group) at which point, if successful, the departed soul would finally arrive home in the safe and benevolent realm of the ancestors (Hicks 2004; Traube 1986). No longer could it torment the living, and in it was invested a power for good (and fecundity), so long as the correct taboos and appropriations continued to be observed (Hicks 2004).

Such occasions, whether private or public, remained, according to our Timorese cultural consultants, a time of intense reflection and self-searching in relation to the cause of death, in which individuals may privately and repeatedly question themselves as to whether some ritual abnegation on their part was somehow responsible. In such instances the symbolic and more concrete reminders of the loss/trauma often appeared to sit side-by-side. This was well illustrated by a young man from the BRR psychotic cohort:

Case BP4

Emilio, a 24 year old single male, was identified by the community as "hanoin barak" and experienced the onset of his first psychotic state during the traditional final mortuary rite, one year after the death of a cousin with whom he was emotionally very close. Although his first two episodes lasted about five days each, significantly his third, most recent episode, had lasted thirty days and was also related to a bereavement—occurring one day after the death of a younger cousin from an unidentified illness.

At the onset of the first episode Emilio had been found holding a machete to his own throat, and when questioned said that people at the mourning celebration had been talking about him and plotting to harm him, despite no one else observing this. Apparently, while he often felt aggressive towards others, the only person (beside himself) he had attempted to harm was his mother who he said he had believed to be a "buang" [approx.. trans. "witch"—from Austronesian-Buli—see below] implicated in the death of his cousin, although no one else in the family held such views. During his last episode he had thrown stones and glass at his mother before the family called the police, following which he was held in a cell for three days. For the remainder of this episode he had appeared very frightened and locked himself in the house, apparently fearful of the police.

To protect him from harm to himself and others, the family acknowledged they had tied him up on more than one occasion as they described him being extremely physically strong in this state needing "eight men to restrain him." In this state he was described as restless and easily distracted, and he would wander around in an agitated state, frequently destroying property in and around the house for no apparent reason. He reportedly slept a great deal less (perhaps three or four hours a night).

Building on this description with the SCID-interview, he was described as talking a lot more and a lot quicker than usual, and sometimes in a nonsensical manner, with no obvious connections between sentences and poorly grounded in reality although his sentences themselves were properly formed and understandable ("you are bad...I am going to have you cut up...I will report you to the police...I am going to fly!"). He also described many physical symptoms associated with the disturbance such as feelings of tension and excitability, alongside the sensation of his heart racing, while he was observed by others, at times, to have "wide frightened eyes" and an observable tremor. When the episode eventually subsided he would reportedly sleep for a good deal of time and on waking reported little memory of the said events. Despite some obvious potential sources of psychological trauma (see Table 2.1*—Emilio) no symptoms of PTSD or inter-episodic depression could be elicited, and he asserted that none of the potentially traumatising events described had caused him significant distress.*

His family asserted that in between these episodes he was reasonably normal except that he was easily angered or upset, sometimes causing him to become vocally aggressive but not physically violent—particularly if asked too many questions or if surrounded by a crowd of people. Indeed during our second interview he had appeared tearful when talking about his young deceased cousin and excused himself from the rest of the interview. During a follow-up visit to discuss treatment with a worker from the new local mental health team, he was home alone and appeared mildly perplexed and suspicious of our presence, although no further evidence of residual psychotic symptoms was evident. He asserted to us that "as far as I know I am normal." His family contended that the cause of his sickness was a "rai nain."

While Emilio was one of only three within the BRR cohort in whom the *fulan lotuk* was not described as a trigger for recurrence, his presentation is consistent with our overall model of symbolically entwined grief and trauma and subsequent ritually-evoked psychotic-presentations, and appears clearly connected with the wider BRR cohort by virtue of *family resemblance* (see Sect. 5.4). Interpreting his inter-episodic perplexity and suspicion towards us is difficult. On the one hand we might see evidence of residual, unsealed dissociative-psychotic symptomatology; on the other this may have been an understandable response to the unsolicited appearance of a *malae* (foreign) doctor asking about a problem he remembers little about.

In relation to his beliefs about this mother, we later read an account of witchcraft from the fellow Austronesian Eastern Indonesian island of Halmahera that the term *buang* (from the Buli language) refers to the living human "carcass" left behind by a parasitic cannibal-witch spirit [Buli: *gua*]. However in doing so the carcass becomes similarly identified as a *human witch*. Local "custom has it that if one fills the abandoned and sleeping body (*buang*) with sharp stones, shards of glass, or broken seashells, the human witch will die" (Bubandt 2014, Chap. 5: The Body of the Witch) along with the parasitic *gua* spirit. The subtleties of this may have been lost in the linguistic and cultural translation of our interview, but it seems likely that a similar belief-system was shared by some in Timor-Leste (either on account of acculturation, diffusion or their shared Austronesian origins—see Sect. 1.3 and also below) and if so, while not necessarily challenging the view that Emilio was psychotic (since his beliefs about his mother were not shared by others), it nonetheless confers an internal logic on his actions that is otherwise not apparent.

Such feelings of intense persecution appear common to brief psychotic presentations in non-industrialised countries (e.g. Jilek and Jilek-Aall 1970) and although common in psychotic presentations in the industrialised world, may playout differently along cultural lines, as we will further explore for Emilio's case, through a psychoanalytic lens, in the following chapter (Sect. 3.1.1, incl. Footnote 4 and 3.1.3).

The Cultural Significance of the *Fulan Lotuk* (New Moon)

While we did not undertake an ethnographic study sufficient to elicit a complete or coherent set of such associations, a lack of a systematic and consistent set of cosmological associations within the Tetum communities in which he participated was previously remarked on by Hicks (2004) leading him to propose that the power of ritual resided within the "realm of performance rather than in that of hermeneutics" (p. 23). Similarly Traube (1986) reflects on her own struggle to piece together mythic narrative fragments in her own efforts to achieve semantic coherence in her understanding of Mambai ritual performance, in which non-verbal elements were seen to be as important as words. Our own evidence suggests that these observations may be at least partly applicable to local understanding and manifestations of mental illness or distress in Timor-Leste and we would agree with Traube (2011) that to propose some overarching semantic logic or framework would likely be more reflective of our own need to create such a coherent cultural world than that of the Timorese-community with whom we worked (cf. Kirmayer et al. 2003; see Sect. 4.2.1)

In line with this it was often difficult to draw out a particular logic of meaning concerning *why* the *fulan lotuk* appeared to be a common and recurrent trigger of psychotic-behaviour in vulnerable individuals—it was simply acknowledged to be part of the natural order of things, although this may also have a reflected a reluctance to share such *lulik* related knowledge. Nonetheless one key cultural consultant, a Timorese mental health worker, with a degree in Philosophy, asserted the significance of this time is less to do with the moon itself, as it is to do with the consequent darkness, left by its absence. Such nocturnal variation in natural light is hard to appreciate in the developed urban setting where many of us now dwell, but in Timor it was striking in both rural areas and urban areas since even in the capital Dili, street lighting was poor and the power supply was not operational during the night. According to this consultant the night/darkness was associated with witchcraft and sorcery. He said at this time the soul of the sorcerer would leave his/her body through an orifice (usually the mouth) and enter that of another, while the potential victim is sleeping and unprotected. The victim may come to know of this through their dreams. The sorcerer's soul is also said to travel and metamorphose—for example into an animal—unseen under the cover of darkness.

Whether our consultant's relatively detailed explanatory model is representative of widely held Timorese beliefs, across different ethnolinguistic groups, is uncertain but would make an important focus of future ethnography. Certainly however there was a striking resonance between our consultant's descriptions and the ethnographic portrayal of witchcraft described above from the regional fellow Austronesian-speaking island of Halmahera,[15] which seemed to confer some logic to Emilio's behaviours. For similar reasons in Timor-Leste, the absolute darkness of the *fulan lotuk* was identified by our consultant as a time ripe for sorcery and witchcraft.

Our model is not reliant on this interpretation, and other symbols and understandings, can as easily be incorporated, although with potential implications for form and content of mental distress. Certainly however we had some further support for the idea of *darkness*, rather than the moon itself, being the key explanatory variable. As one relative of an afflicted individual put it (borrowed for the book's epigraph), "Perhaps because the sky becomes dark, so too people's minds become dark." The suffering of Dores earlier described (see Case BP3), while amplified during the *fulan lotuk*, takes this to the extreme, with symptoms occurring every night fall, and whose content strongly suggest both traumatic and *lulik* dimensions.

Darkness of course, appears to represent, a universal time of increased fear, observed most clearly in children but also in the minds of many adults, as we lack the reassurance and knowledge normally continually bestowed by our eyes. As Harrison (2004) notes, the relationship between darkness and states of mental anguish has been observed throughout history and across cultures and the imagery of darkness is also often used to evoke (and appears to often invoke) dysphoric states of mind. Historically, in the Western cultural tradition, this has a lineage at least as far back as the classical medical theories of Galen (see also Sect. 3.1.2), as Harrison (2004, 594) expounds:

> Melancholy was understood throughout the Middle Ages and Renaissance as being contrary to light and was strongly associated with night, twilight, and darkness… Galen (131-201 AD), wrote of melancholy as not only produced by external darkness, but as also involving an *internal darkening of the mind itself*, giving rise to the fear and sadness [emphasis added].

But darkness however may have brought fear and frightening memories for other reasons too: for even into the post-conflict period at the time of our research, the cover of darkness had been used to strike terror and instability into communities such as Becora, by so called ninjas, groups of youths skilled in martial arts and believed by those we spoke with to be disgruntled in the wake of Timor's independence (cf. Aditjondro 2000). While our local consultant disagreed with this explanation, reasonably asserting that politics and magic were separate realms of explanation, from the perspective of our current framework it seemed possible that

---

[15]In Halmahera, the cannibalistic witch-spirits are similar described as transforming themselves (including similarly into animals) and attacking others at night while they are sleeping (Bubandt 2014).

the connotations of darkness may simultaneously agitate both the symbolic and more concrete associations of terror and trauma.[16]

The question of course is how is this then linked, beyond melancholy, anxiety and dysphoric states, to brief psychotic states of mind? The model of structural dissociation deals with this neatly. An increase in overall emotional distress weakens the effectiveness of dissociative sealing-over—through cognitive and emotional resonance with previous trauma and loss—such that fragmented traumatic memories, emotions and sensations may more easily break through[17] (see Sect. 2.2.1). Such traumatic-resonance may include with culturally connoted, wilfully malign activities (imagined or real) associated with external darkness, feared by some (of witchcraft or "ninja" activity). Such a model becomes more complex when we consider the impact of unconscious agency (see Chap. 3), and sociocultural processes (see Chaps. 4 and 5), but the basic idea of a change in the effectiveness of internal barriers holds (see Sect. 5.3—Fig. 5.1c) and remains compatible with the cultural constructivist position, that such cultural expectations create a context for "acting into" (cf. Pearce 2007; see Sect. 1.7.1).

It is also curious that while beliefs regarding power of unseen forces and spirits such as *rai nain* were well documented by Hicks (2004) and Traube (1986), including as causes of illness and madness, in their ethnographies of Timor-Leste undertaken during the mid to late 1960s, it appears striking that the cyclical phenomena of the *fulan lotuk*, reported so frequently to us, was absent from their accounts of the unforeseen forces impinging on East Timorese daily life. While this might be simply because the anthropology of mental illness lay outside of their focus, Littlewood (1990) points us towards wider ethnographic evidence suggesting that the erosion of traditional ritual practices in some societies is associated with a rise of associated individual symbolic expressions of distress which can be construed as individual unconscious attempts to reproduce the kind of symbolic resolution of intrapsychic and interpersonal tensions previously facilitated through ritual. While we have no evidence or knowledge of the kind of ritual that may have preceded it, given the competing forms of acculturation to which Timor-Leste had been exposed, in particular since Indonesian annexation in 1975 and beyond into

[16]Although culturally, amongst the Mambai at least, the magical and the political, while now considered separate domains, were mythologically understood to have been a unity, and only later subject to division (Traube 2011); we understand that in taking a different position to that of a local cultural consultant we inevitably commit a degree of "interpretive violence" (Bibeau and Corin 1995; cf. Keesing 1995, 220). Nonetheless we understand that the separation of the magic/sacred and political poles makes fundamental cultural sense, and is indeed required. In fact we might be said to do the same through our epistemological division of *deterministic* and *agentic* modes of understanding (Sect. 1.7.1), and in conceptualising sites of intervention—the latter point we will return to in the final section (Sect. 5.5).

[17]Similar ideas were in fact well developed in the models of psychogenic psychosis expounded by Wimmer and other Scandinavian psychiatrists although the intellectual milieu of psychiatry in the remainder of Europe—including Britain and also later in the United States—which had aligned itself with the ideology of biological determinism, prevented ideas of psychogenesis being given due serious consideration (Castagnini 2010; Sass 1992).

the post-Independence period (see Sect. 4.2.3), it seems possible that the phenomenon of transient or exacerbated madness during *fulan lotuk* was either a recent development (arising de novo) or—perhaps more likely—a phenomenon rapidly increasing in frequency and visibility, partly also in the context of widespread trauma. Certainly there has been a shift in Timor-Leste from traditionally bestowed ritual authority to charismatically self-asserted authority (Traube 2007).

Hidden Trauma and Loss

The extent of human rights violations inflicted on the East Timorese under Indonesian rule, and in the wake of the 1999 independence vote, was on such a scale, that on the basis of existing research in post-conflict setting, it would be easy to concur with predictions and observations that a significant proportion of the population would experience substantial mental health burdens associated with post-traumatic reactions (Steel et al. 2009). While our own work indicated that crude questionnaire estimates are likely to significantly overate (by up to two thirds) the prevalence of genuine PTSD in such a population (Silove et al. 2008) and that many people suffering with PTSD–spectrum symptoms may spontaneously improve with the emergence of law and order and consequent greater confidence in personal security (Silove and Steel 2006), others have critiqued the assumptions of Western traumatologists pertaining to the assumed consequences of such violations, in communities in which the meaning and response to such events may markedly differ from our own (Last 2000; Summerfield 1999).

In highlighting *hidden trauma and loss*, in addition to symbolic antecedents and consequences, our intention is neither to minimise the impact of such experience, nor to, a priori, grant it undue weight. The linking of such experiences to the brief psychotic-like reactions described, within the above framework, does, however appear to bring a certain theoretical and pragmatic coherence, although given the almost ubiquitous prevalence of traumatic experiences with the general population, the question as to why some people are more vulnerable to its effects, and why this appears to manifest in different ways in different subjects, remains important to consider. Returning to the concept of hidden trauma then, it was notable how often the experience of any kind of traumatic event was denied, downplayed or simply not associated with (literally *dis-associated* from) the presenting problem. Lack of privacy during interviews, alongside a desire to conform (at least publically) with conventional cultural forms of self-narration, was no doubt an influence here, but might also potentially feed into theorised psychological mechanisms of traumatic amnesia and dissociation—although these may be partly contingent on cultural proscriptions of what can be talked, or even "thought," about.

Case BP5

Marina, a 40 year old female, with a young family, was described by her daughters as "a little 'bulak'" and "pontu." Both she and her daughters described her problems as starting following the death of her paternal uncle and subsequent viewing of his body following which she had "cried all day". The following day she dramatically collapsed on the floor, reportedly hitting her head, and was reported to be unconscious (Tetum: "mate kik"– lit. "little death") for several hours. On wakening she was described as "acting 'bulak' for a whole month" and especially if disturbed by others. At this time she recalled a continuous crawling-like sensation on her face. Subsequently she improved and was able to contribute to subsistence farming, albeit often with little enthusiasm or interest. Additionally her daughters reported outbursts, sometimes two to three times a day, manifesting (according to the SCID) not just as verbally abusive speech but as "disordered speech" (sentences out of context and not meaningfully following one another) and destructive "disordered behaviour" (throwing stones, breaking things). These were in response to various triggers including family disagreement and being left on her own by her daughters, and were notable at the time of the "fulan lotuk."

The experience of a highly traumatic incident emerged, almost incidentally, through the more directive focus of the SCID, in which Marina described witnessing her brother accidentally shoot himself dead while playing with a gun, many years previously. This was an event she "tried not to think about", but was not related either by her or her family in any way to her current presentation. She had some prominent symptoms of both depression and PTSD but these were just subthreshold for a DSM-IV diagnosis although it seems likely that the threshold for one or other would have previously been met. However evaluation of both her psychotic-like symptoms alongside her more non-specific and overlapping symptoms of depression and PTSD (insomnia, irritability, poor concentration etc.*) was complicated by the possible history of head-injury, which may have been sustained after the episode of collapse, even if the collapse itself was of "psychological" origin.*

The above case history illustrates the not infrequently experienced difficulty of obtaining a detailed timeline of events and symptom progression/resolution from past to present, as well as inherent nosological issues with operationalised diagnostic criteria in relation to co-morbidity and diagnostic boundaries (Kendell and Jablensky 2003). In terms of the model developed here, it also highlights both the minimisation of trauma and its consequent entwining in cultural symbols. Cultural proscriptions on what can be talked about, alongside any avoidant disposition or coping style—that might arise or be reinforced by trauma (the avoidant dimension of PTSD, including *overmodulation-numbing* emotional responses (Lanius et al. 2010)—see Sect. 2.2)—would be predicted to be risk-factors for a dissociative response.

Invoking a useful comparison, Kirmayer (1996, 140) draws our attention to the frequency of *susto* or "fright illness" in Central and South America, in which symptoms are often attributed by patients and family members to a "sudden startle, shock or fright". Such dramatic presentations of sudden onset are suggestive of a dissociative aetiology (Steinberg et al. 1994) and indeed "falling-out or blacking out" are linked with dissociative presentations in certain cultural groups, within the DSM-IV-TR Glossary of Culture Bound Syndromes (APA 2000, 900).

In Marina's case both she and her daughter asserted it was the *shock* of seeing her uncle's dead body that gave rise to Marina's subsequent problems. However as Kirmayer (1996, 140) points out "such attributional schemas may complicate efforts to identify traumatic precursors of distress," although of course in Marina's case it might be argued that the emotional and symbolic resonance of seeing her grandfather's dead body connected with her earlier traumatic grief. Our understanding of Marina also supports Csordas et al. (2010) findings that the dual discourses emerging from the SCID and more ethnographic-based interviews, have the potential to complement each other, in furthering our understanding about a particular persons situation and response (see Sect. 1.7.1).

In identifying such trauma as potentially significant we advocate caution, however, so not to give our perspective and explanation privileged status over the family or community. It may be that the family view of her presentation, circumscribes and effectively delimits, the effects of such experience, in an equally or more effective way than Western *psychological* understanding or intervention, better adapted to local culture and context, and about which an individual's distress may often also be read as a commentary (cf. Janes 1995; Skultans 2003). We shall discuss these points further in relation to the *fulan lotuk*. Yet neither should we let our awareness of the differential meanings and responses to such events become an extreme form of cultural relativism, in which we minimise the impact of loss and violation on different communities. Our recent work on "explosive anger as a response to human rights violations in post-conflict Timor-Leste" is a clear indicator of understandable but highly distressing responses to such trauma (Silove et al. 2009), although of course this does not assume the need for interpretation or intervention though a clinical lens.

Table 2.1 highlights the potentially hidden histories of trauma and loss in our index subjects, from within both the BRR and the AOC exacerbation psychotic cohorts combined. It also highlights the symbolic (*lulik*) antecedents of onset and triggers of recurrence, which we have argued to become cognitively and emotionally entwined with the original experience, as well as acting as sources of fear and anxiety in their own right.

Table 2.1 Traumatic and "*lulik*" triggers of onset and recurrence

ID	History of trauma and loss as triggers for onset and/or recurrence	*Lulik* factors as triggers for onset and/or recurrence
BP1 Adriano	Experienced displacement. Endorsed other items on HTQ later denied or minimised. No reporting of loss—but lives with extended family-? parents dead	Family believe strongly in *rai nain* as cause. Recurrence due to *fulan lotuk*
BP2 Ricardo	Fought in Portuguese army against Indonesian invaders. Denies witnessing violence then or subsequently. 2 close family members killed at time of Indonesian invasion (not witnessed)	Visual encounter with *rai nain* but believes broke "contract." Dramatic loss of consciousness while on patrol 1975. Recurrence due to *fulan lotuk*
BP3 Dores	Father killed by Indonesian army in 1984 (not witnessed). Initially described multiple traumas on HTQ but later denied. Nightly hallucinations of soldiers suggestive	Father killed 1984 by military and not "properly" buried and believes she is a possible victim of sorcery. However florid onset of problems not until

(continued)

Table 2.1 (continued)

ID	History of trauma and loss as triggers for onset and/or recurrence	*Lulik* factors as triggers for onset and/or recurrence
	of trauma and linked to fear of darkness? Mother attributes to "broken heart" (*laran kanik*)	2003. Fear of darkness linked with *lulik factors*?
BP4 Emilio	Experienced displacement, separation and "crowds fleeing" but significance downplayed although large crowds may trigger distress. One year post-mortuary rite for close cousin precipitated sudden onset. Subsequent death of another cousin preceded third prolonged episode	Mortuary rite also strongly associated with *lulik* attributions (first episode during this ceremony), and subsequent death of another cousin (preceding third episode) may also have had *lulik* connotations. Family believe *rai nain* implicated
BP5 Marina	1975 witnessed brother accidentally shoot himself dead but subclinical symptoms of PTSD only (unclear if ever met full criteria). Current problems started in 2000 after viewing body of dead uncle. Recurrent distress triggered by being left on own and family arguments	First episode started after viewing of uncle's body (precipitating dramatic collapse)—apparent *lulik* dimension. Believed due to *lulik* problem and recurrence due to *fulan lotuk*
BP6 Julinha	Husband killed by Indonesian military 1975. Problems started after subsequent death of her 2 children in 1997	Recurrence due to *fulan lotuk*
BP7 Luciano	Beaten by militia in 1999 but this was after onset of mental health difficulties	Married but said a *rai nain* made him have sexual relations with another woman 1987 and get her pregnant. Recurrence due to *fulan lotuk*
BP8 Ronaldo	Many symptoms began in 1999 but no history volunteered	Recurrence due to *fulan lotuk*. Claims to be a healer
BP9 Carla	Family report father may have caused it. Recurrence can be precipitated by anger, and becomes angry if does not get own way	One healer suggested cause due to her breaking taboo by touching traditional medicine
BP10 Renata	Lived in jungle as part of female resistance movement but no explicit history given	Encounter with a water sprit (*bai nain*) 1975 when living in jungle—believed to be initial cause. Recurrence due to *fulan lotuk*
CP1 Christiano	Political beating in 1975 but problems started before this. Divorced and possible prior social humiliation may have led to social exclusion and rumination	Unwell for many years. Historically reports seeing a *rai nain* in the form of a snake. Chronic symptoms exacerbated by *fulan lotuk* but also seen as contributing to initial onset
CP2 Fernanda	Temporarily displaced in 1975. Death of 3 children (of 12) but long before onset of problems	Speculation about various possible causes including breaking of *lulik* taboo, and sorcery. Chronic symptoms exacerbated by *fulan lotuk* but also seen as contributing to initial onset

(continued)

Table 2.1 (continued)

ID	History of trauma and loss as triggers for onset and/or recurrence	*Lulik* factors as triggers for onset and/or recurrence
CP3 Eduardo	Family experienced displacement in 1975 due to invasion. Wife and 2 children died while displaced due to sickness	Speculation that onset caused by *rai nain*. Chronic symptoms exacerbated by *fulan lotuk* but also seen as contributing to initial onset
CP4 Lorena	Widowed 1983. Problems attributed to severe head injury 1989—dementia	Obvious physical cause but chronic symptoms exacerbated by *fulan lotuk*

References

Aditjondro, George J. 2000. Ninjas, Nanggalas, Monuments and Mossad manuals: An anthropology of Indonesian State Terror in East Timor. In *Death Squad: the Anthropology of State Terror*, ed. Jeffrey A. Sluka, 158–188. Philadelphia: University of Pennsylvania Press.

Bebbington, Paul E., Dinesh Bhugra, Traolach Brugha, Nicola Singleton, Michael Farrell, Rachel Jenkins, Glyn Lewis, and Howard Meltzer. 2004. Psychosis, victimisation and childhood disadvantage evidence from the Second British National Survey of Psychiatric Morbidity. *The British Journal of Psychiatry* 185(3): 220–226.

Bebbington, Paul, Sarah Jonas, Elizabeth Kuipers, Michael King, Claudia Cooper, Traolach Brugha, Howard Meltzer, Sally McManus, and Rachel Jenkins. 2011. Childhood sexual abuse and psychosis: Data from a cross-sectional National Psychiatric Survey in England. *The British Journal of Psychiatry* 199(1): 29–37. doi:10.1192/bjp.bp.110.083642.

Bentall, Richard P., Sophie Wickham, Mark Shevlin, and Filippo Varese. 2012. Do specific early-life adversities lead to specific symptoms of psychosis? A study from the 2007 The Adult Psychiatric Morbidity Survey. *Schizophrenia Bulletin* 38(4): 734–740. doi:10.1093/schbul/sbs049.

Bibeau, Gilles, and Ellen E. Corin. 1995. From submission to the text to interpretive violence. In *Beyond textuality: Asceticism and violence in anthropological interpretation*, eds. Gilles Bibeau, and Ellen E. Corin, 3–54. Berlin: Walter de Gruyter.

Bovensiepen, Judith. 2011. Opening and closing the land: Land and power in the idaté highlands. In *Land and life in Timor-Leste: Ethnographic essays*, eds. Andrew McWilliam, and Elizabeth G. Traube, 68–86. Canberra, ACT, Australia: ANU E Press. EPUB file.

Bubandt, Nils. 2014. *The empty seashell: Witchcraft and doubt on an Indonesian Island*. USA: Cornell University Press.

Castagnini, Augusto C. 2010. Wimmer's concept of psychogenic psychosis revisited. *History of Psychiatry* 21(1): 54–66. doi:10.1177/0957154X09338086.

Castillo, Richard J. 1994. Spirit Possession in South Asia, dissociation or hysteria? Part 1: Theoretical background. *Culture, Medicine and Psychiatry* 18(1): 1–21. doi:10.1007/BF01384875.

Chung, Man Cheung. 2007. *Reconceiving Schizophrenia*. UK: OUP Oxford.

Csordas, Thomas J., Christopher Dole, Allen Tran, Matthew Strickland, and Michael G. Storck. 2010. Ways of asking, ways of telling: A methodological comparison of ethnographic and research diagnostic interviews. *Culture, Medicine and Psychiatry* 34(1): 29–55. doi:10.1007/s11013-009-9160-4.

Ellenberger, Henri F. 1981. *The discovery of the unconscious: The history and evolution of dynamic psychiatry*. USA: Basic Books.

Evans-Pritchard, E.E. 1976. *Witchcraft, oracles and magic among the Azande*. Oxford: Clarendon Press.

Griffin, M.G., P.A. Resick, and M.B. Mechanic. 1997. Objective assessment of peritraumatic dissociation: Psychophysiological indicators. *The American Journal of Psychiatry* 154(8): 1081–1088.

Guinness, E.A. 1992. Brief reactive psychosis and the major functional psychoses: Descriptive case studies in Africa. *The British Journal of Psychiatry*. 16: 24–41.

Hacking, Ian. 1999. *The social construction of what?*. USA: Harvard University Press.

Hahn, Robert A., and Arthur Kleinman. 1983. Belief as pathogen, belief as medicine: "Voodoo Death" and the "Placebo Phenomenon" in anthropological perspective. *Medical Anthropology Quarterly* 14(4): 3–19.

Hardy, Amy, David Fowler, Daniel Freeman, Ben Smith, Craig Steel, Jane Evans, Philippa Garety, Elizabeth Kuipers, Paul Bebbington, and Graham Dunn. 2005. Trauma and hallucinatory experience in psychosis. *The Journal of Nervous and Mental Disease* 193(8): 501–507. doi:10.1097/01.nmd.0000172480.56308.21.

Harrison, S. 2004. Emotional climates: Ritual, seasonality and affective disorders. *Journal of the Royal Anthropological Institute* 10(3): 583–603.

Hicks, David. 2004. *Tetum ghosts and kin: Fertility and gender in East Timor*, 2nd ed. USA: Waveland Pr Inc.

Hill, Austin, Bradford. 1965. The environment and disease: association or causation? *Proceedings of the Royal Society of Medicine* 58(5): 295.

Janes, Craig R. 1995. The transformations of Tibetan medicine. *Medical Anthropology Quarterly, New Series* 9(1): 6–39.

Janssen, Ian, Lydia Krabbendam, M. Marek Bak, Wilma Vollebergh Hanssen, R. de Graaf, and J. van Os. 2004. Childhood abuse as a risk factor for psychotic experiences. *Acta Psychiatrica Scandinavica* 109(1): 38–45.

Jilek, W.G., and L. Jilek-Aall. 1970. Transient psychoses in Africans. *Psychopathology* 3(6): 337–364.

Johannessen, Jan Olav, Brian V. Martindale, and Johan Cullberg. 2007. *Evolving psychosis: Different stages, different treatments*. Routledge.

Kapferer, Bruce. 1979. Mind, self, and other in demonic illness: The negation and reconstruction of self. *American Ethnologist* 6(1): 110–133.

Keesing, Roger M. 1995. Murder on mount austen: Kwaio framing of an act of violence. In *Beyond textuality: Asceticism and violence in anthropological interpretation*, eds. Gilles Bibeau, and Ellen E. Corin, 209–232. Berlin: Walter de Gruyter.

Kendell, R., and A. Jablensky. 2003. Distinguishing between the validity and utility of psychiatric diagnoses. *American Journal of Psychiatry* 160(1): 4.

Kirmayer, Laurence J. 1996. Confusion of the senses: Implications of ethnocultural variations in somatoform and dissociative disorders for PTSD. In *Ethnocultural aspects of posttraumatic stress disorder: Issues, research, and clinical applications*, eds. Anthony J. Marsella, Matthew J. Friedman, Ellen T. Gerrity, and Raymond M. Scurfield, 131–163. Washington, DC: American Psychological Association.

Kirmayer, Laurence J. 1994. Pacing the void: social and cultural dimensions of dissociation. In *Dissociation: Culture, mind, and body*, ed. David Spiegel, 91–122.

Kirmayer, Laurence J. 2011. Defining and Delimiting trauma-related dissociation: A view from cultural psychiatry. *Journal of Trauma & Dissociation* 12(4): 465–468. doi:10.1080/15299732.2011.570235.

Kirmayer, L.J., D. Groleau, J. Guzder, C. Blake, and E. Jarvis. 2003. Cultural consultation: A model of mental health service for multicultural societies. *Canadian Journal of Psychiatry* 48 (3): 145–153.

Kohen, Arnold S. 2001. The Catholic church and the independence of East Timor.' In *Bitter flowers, sweet flowers: East Timor, Indonesia, and the World Community*, eds. Richard Tanter, Mark Selden, Stephen Rosskamm Shalom, 43–51. Lanham, Maryland: Rowman & Littlefield.

Laddis, Andreas, and Paul F. Dell. 2012. Dissociation and psychosis in dissociative identity disorder and schizophrenia. *Journal of Trauma & Dissociation* 13(4): 397–413. doi:10.1080/15299732.2012.664967.

Lanius, Ruth A., Eric Vermetten, Richard J. Loewenstein, Bethany Brand, J. Christian Schmahl, Douglas Bremner, and David Spiegel. 2010. Emotion modulation in PTSD: Clinical and neurobiological evidence for a dissociative subtype. *American Journal of Psychiatry* 167(6): 640–647. doi:10.1176/appi.ajp.2009.09081168.

Last, M. 2000. Healing the social wounds of war. *Medicine, Conflict, and Survival* 16(4): 370–382.

Lewis-Fernández, Roberto, Alfonso Martínez-Taboas, Vedat Sar, Sapana Patel, and Adeline Boatin. 2007. The cross-cultural assessment of dissociation. In *Cross-Cultural assessment of psychological Trauma and PTSD*, eds. John P. Wilson and Catherine So-kum Tang, 279–317. International and Cultural Psychology Series. Springer. http://link.springer.com/chapter/10.1007/978-0-387-70990-1_12.

Littlewood, Roland. 1990. How universal is something we can call "Therapy"? some implications of non-western healing systems for intercultural work. *Journal of Interprofessional Care* 5(2): 49–65. doi:10.3109/13561829009043447.

Littlewood, Roland. 1996. *Reason and necessity in the specification of the multiple self.* UK: Royal Anthropological Institute.

Littlewood, Roland. 1997. Military rape. *Anthropology Today* 13(2): 7–16.

Litz, Brett T., Nathan Stein, Eileen Delaney, Leslie Lebowitz, William P. Nash, Caroline Silva, and Shira Maguen. 2009. Moral injury and moral repair in war veterans: A preliminary model and intervention strategy. *Clinical Psychology Review* 29(8): 695–706. doi:10.1016/j.cpr.2009.07.003.

McCabe, M.S., and E. Strömgren. 1975. Reactive psychoses: a family study. *Archives of General Psychiatry* 32(4): 447–454. doi:10.1001/archpsyc.1975.01760220059007.

Morrison, Anthony P., Lucy Frame, and Warren Larkin. 2003. Relationships between Trauma and Psychosis: A review and integration. *British Journal of Clinical Psychology* 42(4): 331–353. doi:10.1348/014466503322528892.

Moskowitz, Andrew, Lynn Nadel, Peter Watts, and Jake W. Jacobs. 2008a. Delusional atmosphere, the psychotic prodrome and de-contextualised memories. In *Psychosis, trauma and dissociation: Emerging perspectives on severe psychopathology*, eds. Andrew Moskowitz, Ingo Schäfer, and Martin Justin Dorahy, 2275–2678. Chichester, West Sussex. UK: Wiley-Blackwell. Kindle file.

Moskowitz, Andrew, Ingo Schäfer, and Martin Justin Dorahy (eds.). 2008b. *Psychosis, Trauma and dissociation: Emerging perspectives on severe psychopathology.*. Chichester, West Sussex, Wiley-Blackwell: UK. Kindle file.

Moskowitz, Andrew, J. Read, S. Farrelly, T. Rudegeair, and O. Williams. 2009. Are psychotic symptoms traumatic in origin and dissociative in kind. In *Dissociation and the Dissociative Disorders: DSM-V and beyond*, eds. Paul F. Dell and John A. O'Neil, 864. New York: Routledge.

Muenzenmaier, Kristina H., Azizi A. Seixas, Andres R. Schneeberger, Dorothy M. Castille, Joseph Battaglia, and Bruce G. Link. 2015. Cumulative effects of stressful childhood experiences on delusions and hallucinations. *Journal of Trauma & Dissociation*. doi:10.1080/15299732.2015.1018475.

Nash, William P., and Brett T. Litz. 2013. Moral Injury: A mechanism for war-related psychological Trauma in military family members. *Clinical Child and Family Psychology Review* 16(4): 365–375. doi:10.1007/s10567-013-0146-y.

Niehaus, Isak, Eliazaar Mohlala, Kally Shokane, and Eliazaar Mohala. 2001. *Witchcraft, power and politics: Exploring the occult in the South African lowveld.* Annotated edition. Pluto Press.

Nijenhuis, Ellert R.S., and Onno van der Hart. 2011. Dissociation in Trauma: A new definition and comparison with previous formulations. *Journal of Trauma & Dissociation* 12(4): 416–445. doi:10.1080/15299732.2011.570592.

Ninnemann, Kristi M. 2012. Variability in the efficacy of psychopharmaceuticals: Contributions from pharmacogenomics, ethnopsychopharmacology, and psychological and psychiatric anthropologies. *Culture, Medicine and Psychiatry* 36(1): 10–25. doi:10.1007/s11013-011-9242-y.

Pearce, W.Barnett. 2007. *Making Social worlds: A communication perspective*. Oxford, UK: Blackwell.

Pietrzak, Robert H., and Steven M. Southwick. 2009. The importance of four-factor emotional numbing and dysphoria models in PTSD. *The American Journal of Psychiatry* 166(6): 726–727. doi:10.1176/appi.ajp.2009.09010032. author reply 727.

Read, J., J. Os, A.P. Morrison, and C.A. Ross. 2005. Childhood trauma, psychosis and schizophrenia: A literature review with theoretical and clinical implications. *Acta Psychiatrica Scandinavica* 112(5): 330–350.

Read, John, Paul Fink, Thom Rudegeair, Vincent Felitti, and Charles Whitfield. 2008. Child maltreatment and psychosis: A return to a genuinely integrated bio-psycho-social model. *Clinical Schizophrenia & Related Psychoses* 2(3): 235–254. doi:10.3371/CSRP.2.3.5.

Rorty, Richard. 1989. *Contingency, irony, and solidarity*. Cambridge: University Press.

Ross, Colin A. 2014. Unresolved problems in the theory of structural dissociation. *Psichiatria E Psicoterapia* 33(3): 285–292.

Ross, Colin A. 2008. Dissociative schizophrenia. In *Psychosis, trauma and dissociation: Emerging perspectives on severe psychopathology*, eds. Andrew Moskowitz, Ingo Schäfer, and Martin Justin Dorahy, 8433–8801. Chichester, West Sussex. UK: Wiley-Blackwell. Kindle file.

Ross, C.A., S.D. Miller, P. Reagor, L. Bjornson, G.A. Fraser, and G. Anderson. 1990. Schneiderian symptoms in multiple personality disorder and schizophrenia. *Comprehensive Psychiatry* 31(2): 111–118.

Sakti, Victoria Kumala. 2013. "Thinking Too Much": Tracing local patterns of emotional distress after mass violence in Timor-Leste. *The Asia Pacific Journal of Anthropology* 14(5): 438–454. doi:10.1080/14442213.2013.826733.

Sass, Louis A. 1992. *Madness and modernism: Insanity in the light of modern art, literature, and thought*. New York, NY.: Basic Books.

Scott, James, David Chant, Gavin Andrews, Graham Martin, and John McGRATH. 2007. Association between trauma exposure and delusional experiences in a large community-based sample. *The British Journal of Psychiatry* 190(4): 339–343. doi:10.1192/bjp.bp.106.026708.

Seligman, Rebecca, and Laurence J. Kirmayer. 2008. Dissociative Experience and cultural neuroscience: Narrative, metaphor and mechanism. *Culture, Medicine and Psychiatry* 32(1): 31–64.

Shevlin, Mark, James E. Houston, Martin J. Dorahy, and Gary Adamson. 2008. Cumulative traumas and psychosis: An analysis of the National Comorbidity Survey and the British Psychiatric Morbidity Survey. *Schizophrenia Bulletin* 34(1): 193–199. doi:10.1093/schbul/sbm069.

Silove, Derrick, and Zachary Steel. 2006. Understanding community psychosocial needs after disasters: Implications for mental health services. *Journal of Postgraduate Medicine* 52(2): 121.

Silove, Derrick, Catherine Robina Bateman, Robert T. Brooks, C.Amaral Zulmira Fonseca, Zachary Steel, James Rodger, Ian Soosay, Greg Fox, Vikram Patel, and Adrian Bauman. 2008. Estimating clinically relevant mental disorders in a rural and an urban setting in postconflict Timor Leste. *Archives of General Psychiatry* 65(10): 1205–1212. doi:10.1001/archpsyc.65.10.1205.

Silove, Derrick, Robert Brooks, Catherine Robina Bateman Steel, Zachary Steel, Kalhari Hewage, James Rodger, and Ian Soosay. 2009. Explosive anger as a response to human rights violations in post-conflict Timor-Leste. *Social Science and Medicine* 69(5): 670–677. doi:10.1016/j.socscimed.2009.06.030.

Skultans, V. 2003. From damaged nerves to masked depression: Inevitability and hope in Latvian Psychiatric Narratives. *Social Science and Medicine* 56(12): 2421–2431. doi:10.1016/S0277-9536(02)00245-9.

Spiegel, David, Richard J. Loewenstein, Roberto Lewis-Fernández, Vedat Sar, Daphne Simeon, Eric Vermetten, Etzel Cardeña, and Paul F. Dell. 2011. Dissociative disorders in DSM-5. *Depression and Anxiety* 28(9): 824–852. doi:10.1002/da.20874.

Stampfer, H.G. 1990. "Negative Symptoms": A cumulative trauma stress disorder? *The Australian and New Zealand Journal of Psychiatry* 24(4): 516–528.

Steel, Zachary, Tien Chey, Derrick Silove, Claire Marnane, Richard A. Bryant, and Mark van Ommeren. 2009. Association of torture and other potentially traumatic events with mental health outcomes among populations exposed to mass conflict and displacement: A systematic review and meta-analysis. *JAMA: The Journal of the American Medical Association* 302(5): 537–549. doi:10.1001/jama.2009.1132.

Steinberg, M., D. Cicchetti, J. Buchanan, J. Rakfeldt, and B. Rounsaville. 1994. Distinguishing between multiple personality disorder (dissociative identity disorder) and schizophrenia using the structured clinical interview for DSM-IV dissociative disorders. *The Journal of Nervous and Mental Disease* 182(9): 495.

Summerfield, D. 1999. A critique of seven assumptions behind psychological trauma programmes in war-affected areas. *Social Science and Medicine* 48(10): 1449–1462.

Terheggen, Maaike A., Margaret S. Stroebe, and Rolf J. Kleber. 2001. Western conceptualizations and eastern experience: A cross-cultural study of traumatic stress reactions among tibetan refugees in India. *Journal of Traumatic Stress* 14(2): 391–403. doi:10.1023/A:1011177204593.

Traube, Elizabeth G. 1986. *Cosmology and social life: Ritual exchange among the Mambai of East Timor*. USA: University of Chicago Press.

Traube, Elizabeth G. 2007. Unpaid wages: Local narratives and the imagination of the nation. *The Asia Pacific Journal of Anthropology* 8(1): 9–25. doi:10.1080/14442210601161724.

Traube, Elizabeth G. 2011. Painting the Flag. In *Land and life in Timor-Leste: Ethnographic essays*, eds. Andrew McWilliam, and Elizabeth G. Traube, 117–140. Canberra, ACT, Australia: ANU E Press. EPUB file.

van der Geest, Sjaak and Susan Reynolds Whyte. 1989. The charm of medicines: Metaphors and metonyms. *Medical Anthropology Quarterly*, New Series, 3(4):345–67.

van der Hart, Onno, A. van Dijke, M. van Son, and K. Steele. 2000. Somatoform dissociation in traumatized World War I combat soldiers: A neglected clinical heritage. *Journal of Trauma and Dissociation* 1(4): 33–66.

van der Hart, Onno, Ellert Nijenhuis, Kathy Steele, and Daniel Brown. 2004. Trauma-related dissociation: Conceptual clarity lost and found. *Australian and New Zealand Journal of Psychiatry* 38(11–12): 906–914. doi:10.1111/j.1440-1614.2004.01480.x.

Wallin, David J. 2007. *Attachment in psychotherapy*. New York: Guilford Press.

Widom, Cathy Spatz, Sally J. Czaja, and Mary Ann Dutton. 2008. Childhood victimization and lifetime revictimization. *Child Abuse and Neglect* 32(8): 785–796. doi:10.1016/j.chiabu.2007.12.006.

Chapter 3
Integration with Psychoanalysis and Its Cultural Applications

3.1 Reconstituting Freud

On first reading, the model of traumatic structural dissociation appears to imply a passive "being done to" reaction to catastrophic traumatic stress. In this model trauma is literally inscribed on the mind, as it is the body, leading to mental fragmentation. As generally articulated, there is little consideration of unconscious phantasy[1] or motive, cultural meaning or social response, and perhaps for this reason it has proved attractive to trauma theorists keen on parsimony—arguably lending itself towards a less complicated rendition of people's experiences of trauma and framing the psychomedical response to this. This position might also be seen to be a necessary corrective against the previous dominance of psychoanalysis —with the latter's concomitant preference for exploring internal phantasy as opposed to the significance of external adversity—that may be more in tune with victims *lived experience*.

Yet the universalistic assumptions that underlie models of traumatic structural dissociation fail to adequately consider the role of meaning and social construction evident when examining such experiences. Neither do the social constructionist models, often invoked by anthropologists and transcultural psychiatrists with this focus, escape criticism. As Kirmayer (1993, 170) notes "in each case, the reduction amounts to an unwillingness to acknowledge the ties between symbols and some aspect of the world" and many professionals, service users and carers, feel that constructionist arguments invalidate the psychological impact of trauma in an unhelpful way—for example, as played out over epistemological challenges to the

[1]While there is no accepted definition or usage, and differences between British and American convention, in this work we use the spelling "phantasy" rather than "fantasy" to describe the subject's unconscious ideas and desires, to include, as Isaacs (1948, 81 quoted in Spillius et al. 2011, Chap. 1) puts it, "the psychic representation of instinct." As noted in *The New Dictionary of Kleinian Thought* however, this need not always imply *fanciful deviation* from commonly accepted understandings of interpersonal or material reality (Spillius et al. 2011, Chap. 1).

J. Rodger and Z. Steel, *Between Trauma and the Sacred*,
Cultural Studies of Science and Medicine, DOI 10.1007/978-3-319-24424-2_3

nosological validity of PTSD (see Summerfield 2001 and associated online Rapid Responses).

In this context the re-discovery of Janet, and the work of contemporary attachment theorists and self-consciously termed *relational psychoanalysts* (Mitchell and Aron 1999), might be envisioned as providing much needed redress for the legacy of what Masson (2003) polemically coins, Freud's "assault on truth". Such vehement polarising of positions however precludes any synthesis, and indeed as Ahbel-Rappe (2006) convincingly argues, a more complete and contextual reading of Freud's corpus of work, demonstrates a more nuanced position. Freud acknowledged that external events (including childhood sexual abuse[2]) could be significant, even sometimes *sufficient* (in the absence of other predisposition), to cause severe psychic disturbance, and indeed this was especially clear in Freud's ([1939]2001a, 267–268) later reflections on psychotic delusions, in relation to which he asserted:

> There is not only method in madness, as the poet has already perceived, but also a fragment of historical truth… The vain effort would be abandoned of convincing the patient of the error of his delusion and of its contradiction of reality; and, on the contrary, the recognition of its kernel of truth would afford common ground upon which the therapeutic work could develop.

Similarly suggesting convergence from the other direction, both in theory and practice, advocates of the model of traumatic structural dissociation frequently invoke concepts derived from (or at least consonant with) psychoanalytic theory to complement their understandings of traumatic related symptoms. For example, practitioners working psychotherapeutically with psychotic patients from this perspective, often identify psychotic symptoms as serving an unconsciously agentic and psychologically *defensive* function, while staying within the overarching framework of traumatic structural dissociation (Bacon and Kennedy 2014; Dorahy and Green 2008; Liotti and Gumley 2008; Ross 2008).

Toome (2012), however offers an important critique of such individualised causal modelling of trauma, written particularly with the Timor-Leste situation in mind, pointing to the need to consider wider social, judicial and political responses to trauma, mediating apparent cause and effect. While this and the previous chapter

[2]The psychoanalytic position is often blamed for the failure of late 19th and early 20th Century Western societies to acknowledge the reality of childhood sexual abuse (Castillo 1994; but cf. Gilman 1984). However in relation to Freud's so called "abandonment of his seduction theory" which Masson (2003) argues amounted to a denial of the reality of child sexual abuse, Ahbel-Rappe (2006) cogently demonstrates that a reading of Freud *pro toto* shows that what Freud in fact abandoned was, more specifically, a belief in the *repression of memories* of childhood abuse and their *analytic reconstruction*. Here, we might point out, that contemporary psychologists have also questioned the explanatory value of repression as a concept, instead pointing to models of affect-patterned information processing as an alternative (Kihlstrom 1987, 2005; Seligman and Kirmayer 2008; Kirmayer 1994). Ahbel-Rappe (2006) maintains that Freud continued to acknowledge that childhood sexual abuse may sometimes occur (although perhaps less commonly than he had previously asserted and unhelpfully assigning blame more to older children than adults, who he did not feel had invariably been victims of previous adult sexual assault or seduction).

have been written, with an emphasis on individual psychological processes, we acknowledge that on its own such an account is incomplete, and can only have value if placed in the context of these wider forces, to which we will return in Chaps. 4 and 5.

3.1.1 Basic Mechanisms

In turning to concepts derived from psychoanalysis it is not necessary or appropriate to uncritically embrace the more cross-culturally controversial concepts of psychoanalysis, such as the Oedipus complex,[3] in order to first make use of more basic concepts with explanatory value. In particular, in making sense of the intermittent dissociative-psychotic processes, such as those hypothesized in the current case series there may be value in re-visiting the concepts of primitive defence mechanisms (conceptualised as universal mental processes although no doubt subject to cultural elaboration) described by Sigmund Freud but further developed by others including Melanie Klein in particular (West 2007).

Martindale and Summers (2013) helpfully review these as applied to psychotic symptoms. At centre stage here is the idea of *projection* (see also Lucas 2008)—of aspects of self that are too painful or experienced as too unacceptable to incorporate —onto or *into* others (the latter being an example of *projective identification*). Such a defence seems quite clear in some of our subjects, perhaps most visibly illustrated by two of the most violently disturbed subjects, from the BRR psychotic group, Adriano (Sect. 1.4.2—case BP1) and Emilio (Sect. 2.3.4—case BP4):

Despite the apparent threat of violence when he is psychotic, Adriano's family said the police have not been involved or called directly to any incidents but rather on many occasions Adriano himself has called the police alleging there to be "unrest in the Aldea" although this this was unapparent to others (apart from that caused by Adriano himself).

We might easily read into these behaviours a projection of Adriano's own violent impulses, his desire for containment, and perhaps feelings of guilt (whether past or current), onto others. Indeed Mizen and Morris (2006) have argued that violence itself, is an extension of projective identification—an evacuation of unbearable feelings of the perpetrator—in instances of actual violence, literally *put into* the person–*object*, who might be experienced by the perpetrator as provoking. Although as Mizen and Morris (2006, 71) point out "violence does not beget violence in any simple sense", in the context of past trauma, being a prior victim or witness of literal violent projection, may lead to a need to somehow pass this terror and unwanted violation on to others, in an ultimately unsuccessful attempt to return

[3] Although, at least in Western enculturated persons, the therapeutic framing and subsequent analysis of distorted Oedipal conflicts, has been shown to be of significant therapeutic value in intractable psychotic patients (Jackson and Williams 1994).

oneself to a pre-violated state. There is overlap here with Ferenczi's concept *of identification with the aggressor* (later taken up by Anna Frued) (Howell 2014), itself resembling a dissociative process, in the attempt to find temporary refuge from the wounded part of oneself.

Going beyond projection, Martindale and Summers (2013), describe a range of other basic defence mechanisms, that might be relevant for some of the psychotic cohort, potentially operating simultaneously, or on occasions sequentially. We return to the case of Emilio (Sect. 2.3.4—case BP4):

Emilio was found holding a machete to his own throat at the post-mortuary rite of his cousin, and when challenged by his kinsmen, said that people had been talking about him and plotting to harm him, despite no one else recalling this. He also threatened to report others to the police, and met DSM criteria for pressured and disordered speech. During the interview of family members with the SCID he was described as speaking with no obvious connections between sentences, and poorly grounded in reality, although his sentences themselves were said to be properly constructed. An example included: "You are bad...I am going to have you cut up...I will report you to the police I am going to fly!"

Although an understanding of paranoid ideation or persecutory delusions finds some satisfaction in cognitive models of threat, and the model of traumatic structural dissociation, a psychoanalytic perspective can further compliment this. If our informant accurately recalled his disordered speech, then we can indeed potentially see such simultaneous and sequential defence mechanisms in operation. We appear to start with the *projection* of "badness" into the other (also evidenced in the fuller history of persecutory beliefs and non-shared designation of his mother as a witch: see Sect. 2.3.4) presumably operating side-by-side with the defence of *splitting* in which he sees and presents himself as "good" (further evidenced by his politeness and cooperation towards us as interviewers) despite acknowledging his frequent feelings of aggression towards others and violence towards his mother. Then comes the open acknowledgement of his aggressive feelings, which, as for Adriano, feels in need of containment—possibly by the police (but again threat of police involvement is projected onto others), and perhaps serving simultaneously as addressing his sense of guilt[4] (for his actions towards his mother, for his cousins death, for his own aggression?). Finally he "takes flight" from his feeling altogether, which we might conjecture have become simply too unbearable and threatening to countenance.

"Taking flight" can be seen as a *manic defence* (Ostow 1995) which Martindale and Summers (2013, 126) describe as a response through which "difficult-to-bear

---

[4]Indeed looking at the potential for synergy between culture and psyche, his persecutory beliefs might also be understood as the culturally inverse image of guilt—fitting a context in which the self is not seen as bounded and autonomous, but rather constructed through a social reciprocity and genealogy, which extends into the unseen world. Although his paranoia may also be understandable in the context of a proposed traumatic aetiology (and his fear of the police may have been partly a consequence of his arrest and confinement) persecutory beliefs might also be viewed as a latent cultural possibility of a cosmos where disgruntled spirits are free to roam and hunt the living (cf. Jilek and Jilek-Aall 1970).

feelings of smallness, inadequacy, low self-esteem and shame are commonly unconsciously turned into the opposite." Simultaneously it might be read as a denial of the reality of the body. More generally *thought disorder*, as potentially inferable from the dramatically disordered speech of Adriano and Emilio, and indeed the majority of the psychotic-cohort (see Sect. 1.4.2—Table 1.3) might, in certain instances, be conceptualized as "psychodynamically determined, leading to the breaking up of language and thought that would otherwise have led to ideas with painful or dangerous consequences" (Martindale and Summers 2013, 126).

As illustrated by Emilio, the serial deployment of different defence mechanisms, as the subject seeks different strategies (likely unsuccessfully) to keep painful emotions at bay, may also partly explain the rapidly evolving, *symptom polymorphism*, often seen in transient psychotic states.

Following Bion's (1959) well known paper contemporary commentators also see evidence in psychosis of "attacks on linking" through which the connection between traumatic aspects of reality and psychotic illness is severed (Martindale and Summers 2013). This might certainly be argued for the dramatic and tragic history given for Marina (who had witnessed her sister shoot herself dead but failed to mention this in our interview; see Sect. 2.3.4—case BP5), but as Table 2.1 and the foregoing text should illustrate, the denial or downplaying of trauma was widespread by both psychotically unwell individuals and family collateral historians; no doubt partly reinforced by cultural models that linked mental disturbance to the agency of *rai nain* and other *lulik* forces beyond the human sphere, rather than to the impact of trauma. Indeed the bio-medicalisation of serious mental illness within high income countries, despite the evidence of the powerful social determinants of psychotic experience and illness (see Sects. 2.2.1 and 5.2.6), no doubt serves a similar function, although such processes, intentionally or not, may themselves be partly shaped by political expediency (Taussig 1980). Nonetheless to describe our own dominant medical culture as an "attack on linking" is epistemologically problematic, to describe another's culture as such, is even more so, and loses sight of our ambition to analyse cause and consequence beyond the individual to include the wider community (see Sects. 1.1 and 1.7.2). At such higher levels, apparent "attacks on linking" might be argued to be adaptive for the wider group, at least in terms of the model of political economy currently embraced (or imposed); yet there may be a cost for more vulnerable individuals (Reis 2013).

3.1.2 Symbol Formation

While such political-anthropological critique usefully brings us back to our multi-level analytic agenda, in particular the interaction between culture, unconscious defences, and socioeconomic domains, we need to be cautious of overly superficial readings of culture that have characterised some neo-Marxist analyses (Gaines 1991). For example Bovensiepen (2011) shows that contemporary invocations of *lulik* constitute and articulate complex relationships between people and the land and between each other, and is key in the construction of different cultural identities within Timor-Leste. Obeyesekere (1990) would argue that through such symbolisation, complex "psychoanalytic work" might also be done—perhaps as, or even more, effectively than through a clinical encounter, while also clearly being more consonant with the individuals cultural identity.

Indeed on the subject of symbolism, it is clear that more complex psychoanalytic concepts are implicit in the idea that intrusive flashback-hallucinatory phenomena may be thematic or *symbolic*, not merely representational or echoic of traumatic experiences (Bacon and Kennedy 2014; van der Hart and Wiztum 2008; Read et al. 2005). Indeed in their proposed model of *dissociative psychosis*, van der Hart and Wiztum (2008, 7794) give the example of person developing "hallucinations of being in hell secondarily related to an extreme sense of guilt, during or following a traumatic experience." In Pierre Janet's model of mind—which considerably influenced Carl Jung and Eugene Bleuler's theories of psychological complexes (and their emerging ideas about schizophrenia)—such symbolism might develop by simple association from a primary to a "secondary idée fixes" (the "primary idée" representing the original response to the trauma) (van der Hart and Wiztum 2008; Moskowitz 2008).

As Moskowitz (2008, Endnote 11) points out however, the term *idée,* in this historical psychological context, was much broader than its contemporary usage and instead denoted all "mental elements" including behaviour. Therefore forms of association might include semantic, affective, perceptual and/or visceral resonances —a broad meaning taken up by Bleuler in his concept of "loosening of associations" which became a key concept in his definition of schizophrenia (van der Hart and Wiztum 2008; Moskowitz 2008). This affective dimension of association was particularly taken up by Jung and Bleuler, in their idea of powerful "affect-laden complexes" which operated "much as large galactic bodies drew surrounding mass to them through the force of gravity" and before which other modes of association paled into insignificance (Moskowitz 2008, Sect. 3.4). The example of the association between guilt and the symbolism of hell, given above, clearly has a powerful affective resonance, although the association cannot exist without the cultural–semantic link and we possibly also have a visceral dimension (as in *burning with guilt*[5]).

The importance of symbolism increasingly dawned upon Freud, from his early work on hysteria and in particular in his work on dreams, but was more fully considered subsequently by Melanie Klein who recognised symbolism could have both (and often simultaneously) creative and defensive functions (Spillius et al. 2011). In Freud's understanding of hysteria, even "the absurd idea that causes distress" (such as a notion of hell discussed above) "linked to and symbolically represents the patient's hidden but [more] truly upsetting unconscious idea"

[5]The causes, experience and consequences of guilt (such as going to hell) are of course subject to considerable cultural shaping, in dialectical relationship with more intrapsychic and interpersonal dimensions. Whether the embodied, visceral association of "burning with guilt" has any psychophysiological basis before culture (and upon which meaning is then elaborated) is less clear.

(Spillius et al. 2011, 185). For Klein, representation through symbol, is an attempt to get beyond the anxiety created from relating directly to "primitive experience" and phantasy (that might include desires, fears and conflicts; including in relation to personal and intersubjective bodily experience). She argued, however, that symbols themselves often becomes imbued with the same anxiety and conflict as that which they were intended to represent and displace, leading to a quest for further representation, although in so for as symbols represent aspects of the world, this has a healthy sublimating function, drawing the subject into the world with a thirst for knowledge (Spillius et al. 2011), however this is personally and culturally conceived (scientific, moral, aesthetic etc.).

While it is important to distinguish between the genesis of symbols, their personal meaning, and their cultural associations (Obeyesekere 1984), Klein's ideas, while no doubt influenced by particular Western concepts of self, appear complimentary to anthropological analysis, for example that of Turner (1967). Turner (1967, 30) proposed that public symbols, had both a sensory–emotional and an ideological–social pole, and that the interchange between poles—often in the context of ritual—"converts the [socially] obligatory into the [emotionally] desirable." While anthropologists traditionally have focused on the latter, the importance of the former, including deeply unconscious aspects, is readily acknowledged, although Turner cautions against uninformed forays into this psychoanalytic domain of knowledge.

Obeyesekere (1984), a psychoanalytically-informed anthropologist has however further expounded an understanding of this emotional–unconscious dimension, which as with Turner, challenged previous rigid distinctions between public and private symbols, in arguing that public symbols would cease to meaningfully exist, if they did not have emotional significance, including at an unconscious level, for the individual. While some have construed Obeyesekere's work to assume universal meanings attached to particular symbols (Kunin 2003), in fact he is clear that any hypothesis about cross-cultural similarities in meaning, in relation to a particular symbol, must be tested out in the field. He is also clear that a symbol can only be understood in context, and the same symbol, can have different meanings, within the same culture. For example in our study, the new/crescent moon, referred to as the *fulan lotuk* in the context of transient psychotic disturbance, is also evoked as a symbol of fertility (as a "growing" waxing moon) in the context of annual agricultural rites amongst the Mambai ethnolinguistic group (see Sect. 1.3—Fig. 1.1: Ethnolinguistic map) (Traube 1986).

Returning to Klein, the idea of the symbol itself becoming imbued with conflict and anxiety, is useful for thinking about East Timorese-relationships with important relational symbols, such as their ancestors and *lulik* phenomena (including the associated *fulan lotuk* and *rai nain*), with clearly are seen as having the potential to harm as well as to help. Klein's ideas were expounded and further developed by Hanna Segal, who further differentiated between the formation of the *symbol-proper* and *symbolic-equation* (Spillius et al. 2011). In the former the symbol is understood to represent the object, while in the latter it is *mistakenly identified as the object*. As such where the object is desired it may be used in an attempt to omnipotently deny separation and loss (Spillius et al. 2011), and where the object is feared or hated (which may of course represent a different aspect of the loved object), the subject may feel tormented and persecuted by it. Symbolic equation was seen as characteristic of the paranoid-schizoid position, and has clear application to our understanding of acute psychotic experience, in which experience of "hallucinations" or "delusions" are not usually *understood* to be symbolic or metaphorical by the sufferer, but as intensely and often terrifying real (cf. Kirmayer and Corin 1998).

The concept of the *symbol-proper* also has further anthropological resonance, in particular with Ortner's (1973) work on key symbols in which, elaborating on Levi-Strauss' work, she invokes a subset of key symbols—in particular the *root metaphor*—as particularly useful cognitive tools for thinking with. Klein's clinical work and writing further pointed towards the consequences of a failure to develop symbolic thought, which she felt often underlay childhood autism and psychosis. In an important work, Cashford (2003), a classical scholar, has argued that in agrarian societies lacking industrial light sources, the pre-eminence of the lunar cycle is such to be engrained in the very ecologically-embodied nature of human emotions and thought processes. In other words, returning to Ortner (1973, 1341), the moon is "good to think" with. This is interesting in view of our earlier discussion about the cultural meaning of the *fulan lotuk* tentatively captured by one family member as "perhaps because the sky becomes dark, so too people's minds become dark." This might suggest that the range of *metaphors linking light and thought*, expounded on by Lakoff and Johnson (2003, 48) in Western culture ("understanding is seeing; ideas are light sources"[6] and not least of course the concept of the *Enlightenment*), may have more widespread cross-cultural associations. We have also seen the historical depth of such associations in our own culture, connected to the classical medical theories of Galen (see Sect. 2.3.4) suggesting a similar relationship between external darkness and "an internal darkening of the mind itself" (Harrison 2004, 594). It would of course be helpful if ethnographic work in Timor-Leste could further test out these ideas more widely, in addition to looking for other connections beyond the light-dark metaphor[7].

In light of the above discussion the absence of both literal and "symbolic light" at the time of the *fulan lotuk*, might be partly understood as further *compromising or annihilating symbolic thought*[8]—perhaps particularly in those whose capacity

[6]Examples of "ideas as light sources" given include: "I *see* what you're saying. ... That's an *insightful* idea. That was *a brilliant* remark. The argument is *clear*" and conversely "It was *a murky* discussion...The discussion was *opaque*" (Lakoff and Johnson 2003, 48; italics in original).

[7]Indeed, For Jung (1977) it's waxing and waning stood for the changeability—or corruptibility—of mankind, the latter interpretation taken up by the Catholic church, through the teaching of St. Augustine (Jung 1977), which later became so influential in Timorese culture. It would be interesting to explore ethnographically whether traces of such an idea were evoked through teachings and metaphors used by Catholic priests in Timor-Leste.

[8]Again compare Galen (quoted in Jackson 1986, 42; parentheses in original) "As external darkness renders almost all persons fearful ... thus the color of the black humor induces fear when its darkness throws a shadow over the area of thought [in the brain]" (see Sect. 2.3.4).

for symbolic thought is already compromised[9]—thereby throwing the person back to the primal terror of inchoate, unsymbolised states of mind, or else to the terrifying reality where symbols are experienced as real. The loss of light from the moon may indeed resonate with experiences of traumatic loss more generally. With the transient loss of both the minds symbolic and integrative capacity, such states may be experienced as timeless (West 2007) such that with last vestiges of the waning moon then, the mind is plunged into what might feel like an endless darkness—only for the early waxing moon, to bring some sense of restored time and re-ignition of the symbolic (and thereby distance from, or ability to seal-over, the terror of the experience). While a full discussion is beyond the scope of the present work, we might contrast this with the cultural connection between madness and the full-moon in the Euro-American cultural tradition. [10]

In her analysis of autistic and psychotic children Klein discovered rudimentary forms of symbolism (often behaviours) that she successfully helped the children build upon. In an analogous manor, we shall argue that the social response and cultural meanings given to madness in Timor-Leste appear to have a similar constructive function of symbolic scaffolding and enhancing communication, delimiting the temporal scope and impact of such disorder (see Sects. 3.1.4, 4.2.1 and 4.2.2). In other social or cultural contexts however, characterised by a more destructive and harmful "malignant social positioning," poorer outcomes might be predicted (cf. Kitwood and Bredin 1992; Sabat 2006—see Sects. 4.2.2 and 5.2.2).

---

[9]This is a difficult to assess cross-culturally. Certainly in at least two persons from the BRR cohort (interviewed inter-episodically when well—BP4, Emilio and BP10, Renata: see Sect. 2.3.4 incl. Table 2.1) we were struck by what from our own perspective appeared to be a *concreteness of thought*, possibly indicative of impaired symbolic capacity (Pestalozzi 2003). However this might also be explainable by difficulties with concept translation, lack of formal education and apparent amnesia for the events in question. Impaired symbolic capacity might itself be secondary to past overwhelming trauma (see Sect. 4.1.1).

[10]*Consistent* empirical evidence of an association between the moon and psychotic reactions or exacerbations is lacking in Western societies (McCrae 2011; see also Sect. 5.4), but since streets and homes in high-income countries are often flooded with electric lights, alongside the decline of the power of myth in our secular age (Obeyesekere 1984, pt. 3: Myth Models; see Sects. 4.1.1 and 4.2.1), any looping effect (Sect. 1.7.2) between cultural attributions regarding the lunar cycle and changes in mental state and behaviour is likely to have been significant weakened. As Sass (1992) notes however in his monumental *Madness and Modernism*, sometimes an association might be at the level of analogy rather than causality. Of course, under the right conditions, our thesis would suggest that such a metaphor may become both trigger and context to "act into" (cf. Pearce 2007; see Sect. 1.7.1), if symbolically resonant with individual experience (see Sect. 4.2.1). However cultural symbols derive meaning not from absolute properties but from their cultural interpretation, and relation to other symbols. Therefore although we might conjecture that the full-moon in pre-industrial societies might have made an apt metaphor for the *excess of feeling and thought* characteristic of a manic-episode, a full but waning moon might, as with the new moon in Timor-Leste, be a symbol of loss after its peak (cf. Silva 2008), as in the saying from *The Witch of Edminton*, (quoted in McCrae 2011, 51) "When the moon's in the full, then wit's in the wane." Similarly the new moon and early waxing crescent can be a symbol of growth to come, and indeed is invoked in a different context, amongst the Mambai of Timor-Leste, in their "rites of transition" at the end of the dry season (Traube 1986, 156).

3.1.3 Phantasy Verses Reality

In much psychoanalytic discussion about symbol formation the underlying theme appears to be about how phantasy (as expressions of unconscious drives, wishes and conflicts) interacts with realty, and through which a patient's symbolisations are formed or symptoms become manifest in compromise arrangements. Implicit here is an elevation of the status of "psychic reality" to a least equal footing to—if not, for many analysts, higher footing than—that of external reality. In the context of real past trauma and human rights violations, Adriano and Emilio's threats to call the police (see earlier Sect. 3.1.1) might be understood as a blurring of inner and outer realities, manifest as "confusion about who is bad and who deserves to go to jail" but complicated "in the face of constant inner condemnation" (Jackson and Williams 1994, 40) and persecutory guilt.

While we have earlier cautioned against the uncritical translation of more complex, controversial and arguably more culturally specific ideas, such as the Oedipus Complex, to Timor-Leste, both psychoanalysts and anthropologists have taken its question seriously, as applied to clinical (including psychotic) and ethnographic, non-Western, populations. Various revisions have been offered since Freud, taking into account changing clinical insights and cultural understandings, including less emphasis on erotic dimensions and more on negotiating multiple attachments and power, commentaries on patriarchy, capitalism and Western idealised concepts of the autonomous self, different cultural sublimations or elaborations, inversions and partial forms, and whether the father is real or symbolic—the latter, depending on the forms of kinship organisation and associated patterns of descent and post-marriage residence (Bhugra and Bhui 2002; Obeyesekere 1990; Parsons [1964]2010).

For Timor-Leste, lacking further ethnographic data we do not have enough information to confidently comment although Traube (1986) describes important mythological antecedents to customs around sex and the incest taboo amongst the Mambai. More directly supporting this line of inquiry Hicks (1984, 102–105) describes an evocative folk-tale recounted by the patrilineal and patrilocal Tetum from the eastern district of Viqueque (see Sect. 1.3—ethnolinguistic map) involving filicide, resurrection of the son, and father-son conflict (symbolised in a "cock fight[11]"), taken to the death, with the eventual usurping of kingly power by the son. Indeed this tale was included in the collected volume of global folk tales in support of the theory, Oedipus Ubiquitous (Johnson and Price-Williams 1996). However, even where more clearly present within certain culture groups, the clinical relevance for a given individual, needs to be determined, and such hypothesis probably need

[11]In light of the double meaning ascribed to the word "cock" in English, it is of interest in the context of this discussion about the Oedipus complex, that the compound Tetum words for penis and cockerel share the same root, *manu*, translated as a bird or chicken. Additional suffixes narrow or transform meaning such that cockerel is denoted *manu aman* (chicken + male) and penis is *manu oan* (chicken + young).

to be understood within a more general framework of symbolic healing (Dow 1986), and an appreciation of the theoretical persuasion of the healer in question (Bhugra and Bhui 2002).

Additionally, we need not necessarily embrace all Oedipal premises and elements to acknowledge the impact of the complex intrafamilial power dynamics and attachments apparent in all families, and the theory itself provides some striking illumination to the question of what the consequence might be when *phantasy meets reality*. What for example of a young boy who might unconsciously phantasize a wish to usurp his father, and whose father is then killed in combat, and who, culturally and economically, may be thrust prematurely into the position of being "man of the house" within a context, common in Timor-Leste, where extended family networks may have been fragmented or destroyed? A risk-factor for terrifying psychotic omnipotence and persecutory guilt? If so might this become further reinforced by a belief that *lulik obligations* have been neglected (e.g. if the father was "wrongly" killed, improperly buried or not subject to appropriate post-mortuary rites—see Sect. 2.3.3—Case BP3)—although equally such beliefs and associated practices may offer a path towards symbolic and emotional restitution (see Sect. 5.5), in addressing painful psychic realities at a greater degree of symbolic remove (cf. Obeyesekere 1990).

3.1.4 Levels of Psychic Organisation and Representation

Moving to a further level of complexity, in an important paper Hirsch and Hollender (1969) anticipated more recent attempts to reconcile psychobiological and social theories of dissociation in their attempted rehabilitation of the term "hysterical psychosis." They proposed that psychotic-like presentations, in persons of "hysterical character" (to whom they attributed a distinctive cognitive and perceptual style not dissimilar to current concepts about dissociative proneness; cf. Seligman and Kirmayer 2008) may arise in a process analogous with somatic-conversion, but in which *lay notions of madness* become appropriated in the place of the neurological symptoms traditionally associated with the disorder. They also proposed that because such behaviour was in essence goal orientated (albeit unconsciously—presupposing psychodynamic concepts of ego integrity and *successful* repression), and generating a constructive social response, that such behaviour might be seen as tacitly culturally sanctioned and that this in turn shaped their form.

Through this lens, they also differentiated the "psychotic-like" behaviour of dissociative-conversion, from what they understood, *still within a psychodynamic paradigm*, as "true psychotic states"—the latter understood as a de-compensated state of ego-disintegration resulting from an overwhelming of dynamic defences. This is the quintessential Freudian model of psychosis involving *failed repression*, and as such is not presumed to have a psychologically or socially adaptive function for the individual. This contrasts with the *compensated-state* described above, in which successful repression of culturally forbidden desires and drives (for Freud Oedipal sexuality and aggression) is assumed, and which for the "hysteric" (and "hysterical psychotic") are theorised as *symbolically resolved*, and kept from conscious awareness, in the formation of somatic (or in our study, psychotic-like) conversion symptoms.

Whether such a form of psychosis—reflecting an absolute failure of repression truly exists (at least for long)—or whether it might be more fruitful to think of repression as a matter of degree, is an important question. A common example often given of failed repression is that of wish-fulfilling ego-syntonic hallucinations, often of a grandiose nature, theorised as infantile attempts to mitigate desire (Eigen 2004). They are understood as psychotic in so far as they are mistaken for reality (Segal's symbolic equation—see earlier Sect. 3.1.2). More often than not, however, a failure of repression—traditionally viewed as a "neurotic defence"—would be assumed to give way to the more primitive (and in some cases psychotic) defences outlined earlier (see Sect. 3.1.1). Sometimes the "correct" (and culturally appropriate) formulation might be hard to make. For example, the violence seen in some psychotic states, might be understood to be direct expressions of underlying, *un-repressed* drives against a hated or desired object, but equally (as discussed earlier) could be thought of an extreme extension of projection or projective identification, in which intolerable feelings are literally "put into" the other (often inducing reciprocal violent feelings in the other).

Less directly, ego-dystonic abusive auditory hallucinations or paranoid beliefs, might be understood as a disavowal of the persons own aggressive feelings, projected out onto a disembodied external "voice", specific person or people in general. Relationships of such experiences with trauma are again complex and often polemical. Speaking against the psychoanalytic position we can see how some might see such ideas as potentially blaming the victim for being the locus of aggression, rather than acknowledging paranoid thoughts and persecutory voices as articulating a sense of violated trust in the world or as fragmented or symbolic representations of actual events as earlier discussed (Sect. 2.2.1). On the other hand, the psychoanalytic position, acknowledges a person's response to trauma (which may include rage and aggression) can be as problematic as the event itself, and a person, for example, who previously saw themselves as peace-loving, might be as afraid of their own aggression, as they are of others, and therefore disavow it. Both could be true in the same individual. It also seems likely that the actual experience of real past trauma makes what previously seemed only a possibility of violence (in imagination), frighteningly real (in both self and other), such that it might seem (and indeed happen) to burst into existence at the slightest provocation (cf. Silove et al. 2009).

Connected to this, how such Freudian concepts of repression interface with the Janetian derived model of structural-dissociation (see Sect. 2.2) is also important to consider. While we have discussed some aspects of their different emphasis on reality and phantasy, there is also the juxtaposition of two different models of what is *non-conscious*—metaphorically Freud conceived of this *layered horizontally* (his "topographical model") with decreasing levels of conscious availability as one moved from conscious awareness through the "preconscious" to "the unconscious" (Castillo 1994). In contrast Janet and his followers however, conceived that consciousness could be divided *vertically* into compartmentalised self-states (Moskowitz 2008), termed by Janet "the subconscious" but perhaps more depictively evoked by Morton Prince's image of "co-consciousness" (Castillo 1994, 6).

Whereas Freud's unconscious was comprised solely of "unacceptable" phantasies, conflicts and impulses, actively repressed from conscious awareness in a dynamic process, for which there was a psychic *energetic cost*, co-consciousness was understood to contain both painful real memories and affects, as well as non-distressing happier ones, that clustered together with other material through the process of association described earlier (Castillo 1994; Moskowitz 2008). For Janet then the subconscious is the repository of *split-off* (rather than repressed) affects, memories, associations and representations of *real* abuse and trauma—that, in a de-compensated state, break-through to conscious awareness, overwhelming and de-orientating the self, leading to a psychotic states of mind. In both models of "true" dynamic psychosis however, the barrier between the conscious and unconscious/subconscious mind is breached and consciousness overwhelmed. At the level of ideal-types, the key difference lies in whether or not the fragmented experiences entering conscious awareness are felt to have their roots in reality (Janet) or phantasy (Freud). [12] As with repression however, dissociative splitting-off, is likely to be a matter of degree, rarely completely successful, but rarely wholly defeated (again, at least for very long).

Since even in florid states of psychosis, symbolic manifestations of psychic-content are usually apparent (albeit perhaps requiring decoding[13]), this

---

[12]In fact, Freud did acknowledge the impact of external traumatic experience, particularly in his early work but also in later work, including his account of the genesis of delusions (see Sect. 3.1). In his earlier work, referring to "traumatic neuroses" Freud ([1917]2001b, 274–275) wrote that "These patients regularly repeat the traumatic situation in their dreams; where hysteriform attacks occur that admit of an analysis, we find that the attack corresponds to a complete transplanting of the patient into the traumatic situation. It is as though these patients had not yet finished with the traumatic situation, as though they were still faced by it as an immediate task which has not been dealt with." However, notwithstanding such acknowledgements, throughout his writings Freud generally privileged intrapsychic realities over external ones.

[13]With the development and publication of DSM-III in 1980 mainstream psychiatry moved away from an understanding of mental distress informed by social science and psychoanalysis (Wilson 1993), and thereby questions of meaning. While DSM-III and its successors (now up to DSM-5) avouch to be atheoretical, as Gaines (1992, 3) has shown, a deep rooted "ethnobiological essentialism" in fact permeates the texts, and contemporary dominant biological approaches to psychosis continue to eschew questions of meaning as irrelevant. Indeed, the notion that psychotic phenomena were beyond understanding, is often attributed to Karl Jaspers, however as Hoerl (2013) has clearly shown, a close reading of Jasper's *General Psychopathology* and related publications, suggests Jasper's attempted to *understand* psychotic phenomena (which he differentiated from *causally* explaining). This included an interest in what he termed *true reactive psychosis* (German: *echte reaktive Psychose*) which had some influence on the Scandinavian school (Castagnini 2010, 55). He did however acknowledge limits of understanding, in particular, where psychotic symptoms were not readily understandable from prior psychological states, for example, as in passivity phenomena (Hoerl 2013). We would argue however that in some

would imply not just the interaction of phantasy and reality,[14] but the personal with the cultural, and suggests psychological processes of defensive transformation have not wholly collapsed. While failure of repression or splitting-off have the potential to lead to a more complete psychological state of integration, this side-steps the question as to why repression or splitting-off occurred in the first place—the roots of which may be a product of personal history (including trauma and phantasy) and possibly biological inheritance, or more immediate and ongoing social and cultural factors, for example relating to familial proscription, social stigma or taboo.

Furthermore such rudimentary symbolism (even if manifest simply at the level of behaviour and requiring de-coding) will generate a social response that has the potential to further contain and productively expound and transform symptoms and distress (or else negate and provoke; see Sects. 4.2.2 and 5.2.2). While Wiztum and van der Hart (2008) criticise Hirsch and Hollender's (1969) revised model of "hysterical psychosis" for incorporating cultural sanctioned behaviour and on account of their differentiation of dissociative–*conversation* psychosis from *true* dynamic psychosis, on the grounds that it conflates genuine dissociation with consciously motivated fabricated illness and malingering, such a position is based in our opinion, on the faulty view that within the myriad presentations of psychosis there is no room for a spectrum of *greater or lesser psychic organisation* and that

(Footnote 13 continued)

instances an apparent lack of understanding may be simply due to a lack of sufficient personal and contextual information; in other instances breakdown in inference from prior psychological states may be on account of mental leaps mediated by unconscious processes, particularly the more primitive psychodynamic defence mechanisms earlier discussed (Sect. 3.1.1), that do not readily lend themselves to empathic understanding by non-psychotic individuals. In any case, there is a long history of resistance to DSM's influence, amongst which we would include transcultural psychiatric (e.g. Jenkins and Barrett 2004—edited vol.), psychoanalytic (e.g. Jackson and Williams 1994; Lucas 2008) and genuine phenomenological (e.g. Humpston 2014; Sass 1992) approaches to psychosis, alongside much detailed ethnographic work (for a list of recent works see Hopper 2008) that have attempted to illuminate understanding and meaning in psychotic phenomena. It obviously also includes the work of the so called anti-psychiatrists, such as R. D. Laing, who were an important inspiration for a new generation of critically minded psychiatrists (e.g. Bracken et al. 2012; Thomas et al. 2004). Such approaches strive for "thick description" and tend to draw on sociological, interpretative and cultural phenomenological approaches, alongside systemic and psychoanalytic thinking, in order to re-position questions of meaning and context as a central concern. While in most countries such critical voices have remained subaltern, in France (Vallée 2011) and until recently in Scandinavia (Castagnini 2010), resistance has been more institutionalised within national frameworks of practice including alternative diagnostic schemata, and spawning alternative therapeutic approaches, attending to context and meaning—an important example being the intensive, network-systemic Open Dialogue and trauma-informed approach to new onset psychosis in Finland (Seikkula et al. 2011) that has published exceptional and provocative outcomes, and to which we will return in later discussions in the final chapter.

[14]Indeed, as explicated earlier (see Sect. 2.3), the laying down of memories itself is always mediated through personal, social and cultural filters (even when spilt-off) and invariably re-worked over time. There is therefore no original primary experience or memory on which to call upon, untouched by social and cultural processes (Dennett 1993).

the cultural shaping of dissociative-conversion processes cannot happen outside of the subject's awareness (even if secondary gain is apparent to the observer).

Such disagreements are characteristic of the wider tension between those who view dissociative phenomena as wholly reflections of a deterministic traumatic fragmentation of an individual's constitutive psychological make-up and those who emphasize the importance of *personal agency* (albeit potentially at an unconscious level) and *social role*, that leaves no room for potential synthesis, such as with Hacking's (1999) model of "interactive kinds" (see Sect. 1.7.2). We will go onto argue that it is particularly fragmented selves that may be most susceptible to cultural templates and social-roles that may give a fragmented self some form. This may not be nuanced self-conscious cultural positioning and interpretation, but more concrete less conscious grasping of form (see Sect. 4.2.1), that may be even more fraught in a culture, in which traditional forms are subject to erosion and attack from competing forces (see Sect. 4.2.3). Cultural symbols and behavioural scripts, with their public/social and private/emotional poles (Obeyesekere 1984; Turner 1967—see Sects. 3.1.2 and 4.2.1), are well placed to mediate between these internal and external forces impinging on the psyche.

3.2 From Individual to Relational Models: Developmental Considerations

If we accept the interactional model of structural dissociation and internal phantasy, mediated by symbolic representations, as one possible pathway through which trauma may contribute to the genesis of psychotic symptoms, we still need to ask ourselves why certain individuals appear more vulnerable to such an outcome (cf. Spauwen et al. 2006), however this is clearly multifactorial and difficult to predict prospectively. Certainly trauma appears to impair the contextual embedding of memory in individuals with clinically-related symptoms. This has been well described in classical-PTSD but may be even more prominent in a dissociative-PTSD subtype (Lanius et al. 2010), and as such has provided a useful model for thinking about psychotic-symptoms as dissociative in origin (see Sect. 2.2.1).

The nature of trauma is also significant. Predictably perceived *severity* and *chronicity* of trauma appear key predictors of dissociation, but a single episode of trauma, may give rise to recurrent dissociative-experience, particularly if associated with *peritraumatic dissociation* at the time of the traumatic-insult—which is itself linked to higher perceived levels of threat (for example, if experienced as life-threatening) (Griffin et al. 1997; Lanius et al. 2010). This might be because peritraumatic dissociation interferes with the encoding of traumatic and wider contextual memory at the time of the event, or because once established as a potential coping mechanism, it is available for repeated use, in response to triggers or intrusions of the original trauma, or in the face of further adversities. All of these factors are clearly relevant to the protracted and systematic campaign of terror waged by the Indonesian military and sponsored militias against the East-Timorese population (cf. Aditjondro 2000).

Trauma earlier on in the life-course, and in childhood, also appears to be a greater risk factor for both dissociation and the ability to dissociate (Lanius et al. 2010; Seligman and Kirmayer 2008), and indeed the majority of the studies exploring links between psychosis and trauma documented childhood trauma and maltreatment as risk factors,—albeit later compounded by further adult trauma and adversity (Read et al. 2005). The findings are increasingly being replicated across different cultural groups, although what counts as traumatic, even in relation to bodily-trauma, may have some cultural-variability (Lewis-Fernández et al. 2007). Contiguous with earlier Scandinavian models of psychogenic-psychosis,[15] developmental models generally propose a dual or multi-stage model of problematic development, with an initial traumatic sensitisation, amplified by later life trauma and adversity, which may clearly help to explain why for some trauma gives rise to simple PTSD, while for others more complex dissociative states, and greater degrees of fragmentation are apparent (Cloitre et al. 2009; Liotti 2006).

Whether genetic factors have a direct role in predisposition to dissociation is uncertain (Becker-Blease et al. 2004) although pre-existing personality traits, such as fantasy-proness and capacity for absorptive experience—while potentially contributing to healthy and creative functioning in many contexts—may be risk-factors for dissociative-responses in the face of trauma and adversity (Seligman and Kirmayer 2008). It is therefore also of interest that some leading contemporary geneticists are arguing that particular genes may be adaptive or harmful depending on the wider environmental or interpersonal context. Of particular relevance to our work is research indicating that specific dopamine-receptor genes (additionally implicated in psychosis) may influence the risk of disorganised attachment (a likely developmental precursor of dissociation—see discussion below) in response to unfavourable caregiver environments yet may confer benefit, above-and-beyond the norm, when exposed to a more favourable caregiving (Belsky et al. 2009 on "plasticity genes").

The relationship between childhood and dissociative tendencies, however, is also complex with some arguing that children generally have naturally greater dissociative abilities that may have become lost in cultures where dissociative experience is devalued or pathologised (Seligman and Kirmayer 2008). Certain cultures also appear to foster dissociative abilities in children through social learning. In Timor-Leste definite learnt processes of dissociation where in operation. The most notable we observed was the process of funeral wailing ("keening") by young children, who could be seen to switch this outward manifestation of their sorrow *on and off* at will—alternating with laughter and play—in a process of

[15]Captured by the concept of "catathymia" (a term originally coined by the Swiss psychiatrist W. M. Maier in 1912) and invoked by both Wimmer ([1916]2003) and Faergeman (1963) in their classic works; Castagnini (2010, 55) outlines this as "the process of sensitization whereby memories of past experiences are recollected by events thematically related to them, provoking abnormal (idiosyncratic) reactions."

socialisation and mimicry of their adult counterparts. Adults assumed a more genuine and involuntary demeanour but could nonetheless also quickly curtail their keening in response to social cues, such as arrival of newcomers or offering of prayers. Their grief is of course undisputed—permission for its spontaneous "involuntary" expression is however subject to a considerable social conditioning yet such social contexts provide a space into which real feeling persons may act into[16] (cf. Pearce 2007; see Sect. 1.7.1). Whether innate or acquired, in situations of trauma or maltreatment however, children may turn to such dissociative abilities as a coping mechanism that becomes reinforced over time (Seligman and Kirmayer 2008), and this assumes a developmental trajectory from the adaptive to the maladaptive (Kirmayer 2011).

An underlying theme here is dissociation as a relational phenomenon and as such the over reliance of psychoanalytically minded anthropologists on *intrapsychic* explanations of dissociative presentations has been subject to critique and more *intersubjective* models of psychic life put forward as useful alternatives and arguably providing a better fit with the relational assumptions privileged by social anthropologists (Hollan 2012; Lambek 2003). In particular the findings of contemporary *Attachment Theory* researchers have been used to critique and revise more traditional psychoanalytic assumptions (Fonagy 2001; Holmes 2001) giving rise to Relational Psychoanalysis (Mitchell and Aron 1999). Attachment Theory proposes that *internal working models* of concurrent and prospective relationships are grounded in early infantile relational experiences with primary caregivers, and that different *attachment strategies* may be adaptively employed by infants and children, to adaptively cope with differing relational contexts, ranging from the sensitive and reflective, to neglectful or traumatic (Hesse and Main 2000). Robust empirical findings from Attachment Theory have found a startling continuity in Attachment Strategies between early life and adulthood (Hamilton 2000) and across generations (Benoit and Parker 1994).

While the concept of attachment demands further cross-cultural critique, it is of interest that many of the key original tenants of the theory were borne out of a study of children in Uganda, and at the behavioural level at least, the premise is argued to have universal applicability, as long as: cultural variations in how attachment seeking behaviours are displayed is acknowledged (as influenced by differential cultural meanings and expectations), that contextual and ecological factors are considered (including what is adaptive under those conditions), and that the focus of relationships is extended beyond the maternal-infant dyad, to a wider network of caregivers and kin (van IJzendoorn and Sagi-Schwartz 2008). While the assessment of *attachment states-of-mind* in adults relies on the analysis of narrative structure rather than behaviour, given the observed ubiquitous centrality of narrative in the cultural construction and articulation of human experience, including the relevance of narrative to dissociative phenomena (cf. Kirmayer 1994), it seems likely that

[16]Bourdieu (1992, 73) approaches this from the obverse: "The body believes what it plays at: it weeps if it mimes grief."

links between early attachment experiences and later narrative structure and style will be found to have relevance across cultures, as long as similar nuanced sensitivity to linguistic convention, cultural meaning, ecological niche and cultural models of the ideal self are given due respect and consideration, although so far cross-cultural studies in adult attachment narratives have been limited to Japan (cf. van IJzendoorn and Sagi-Schwartz 2008).

While work exploring the implications of networks of caregivers, beyond the mother-infant dyad, is itself in its infancy (van IJzendoorn and Sagi-Schwartz 2008), and Western cultural ideals of adult autonomy are an embedded unhelpful core assumption of the model (Keller 2012), its wider implications in terms of understanding trauma and dissociation are clear. Attachment theory in particular suggests that children trapped in unescapable abusive relationships with their primary adult caregivers will experience something of a double-bind, or "fright without solution," (Hesse and Main 2000, 1106) caught between the evolutionary imperative to stay close to the caregiver for food and protection, while trying to avoid further episodes of maltreatment. This impasse can lead to rapid oscillation between approach and avoidance, freezing, and unusual postures or facial expressions when in the proximity of the "caregiver" (Hesse and Main 2000). Classified as a *disorganised attachment* strategy it is oddly reminiscent of classic catatonic behaviours sometimes seen in severe psychosis such as ambitendency, motoric immobility, posturing, and grimacing[17] (Casher and Bess 2010), which Moskowitz (2004) argues may themselves represent evolutionarily wired fear-based responses. A disorganised attachment strategy in childhood has been empirically demonstrated to be a significant risk factor for later dissociation, perhaps because the self-psychobiological subsystems implicated in structural dissociation never find coherent integration in the first place(cf. van der Hart et al. 2004).

While accepting that cultural definitions of maltreatment are subject to some cross-cultural variability (Korbin 1991), there is growing international recognition of the reality of childhood maltreatment in non-Western settings (Finkelhor and Korbin 1988), and Timor-Leste is no exception to this ('Annotated Bibliography of Child and Forced Labor Information' 2009; Tang 2002). Family tensions would of course be predicted to dramatically increase in periods of chronic hardship and adversity characterising a conflict situation. Add to this the direct witnessing or experiencing of violence or other types of intentional harm by family members and we might not be surprised that other family members, including children, could become subject to the cycle of further violent projection within the family (Rees et al. 2013).

Of likely even greater significance however for countries such as Timor-Leste, is the recognition that *unresolved caregiver grief and trauma*, are in themselves significant predictors of disorganised infant attachment, and that the genesis of

[17]The meaning and resonance of some of these terms is self-evident. Perhaps less evidently *ambitendency* is described as "appearing 'stuck' in an indecisive, hesitant movement" and *posturing* refers particularly to the maintenance of often unusual and uncomfortable postures for extended periods (Casher and Bess 2010, 37). Catatonia can also be seen in the presence of organic disease affecting the brain.

disorganised attachment states of mind has been empirically demonstrated to be mediated not just by *frightening* caregiver behaviour, but also by *frightened* caregiver behaviour (Hesse and Main 2000; Liotti 2006)—a likely common consequence of living under conditions of conflict and terror. Although it is important to acknowledge that certain local ecological factors, incorporating culture and context (such as the availability of extended kinship networks, meanings given to trauma, political processes, neighbourhood cohesion and collective competence) may buffer individuals within a given community against some of the deleterious effects of trauma, it is equally important to ask under what conditions collective and individual resilience may be overwhelmed (Hoshmand 2007)? In particular in a country afflicted with loss and trauma to the extent seen in Timor-Leste, where up to a third of the population is estimated to have died across the 25 year period of Indonesian rule often associated with periods of severe violence and repression, community and kinship resources and support would likely have been overwhelmed, at least for periods of time, and in certain communities—particularly given such acts of commission, often co-occurred alongside the induced omission of other basic tenets of human security, such as shelter, food and medicine (Silove et al. 2009). Multiple and cumulative adversity poses a particular risk for disorganised attachment and a wide range of later mental health difficulties, including psychosis (Read et al. 2005; Shaw and Vondra 1993; Turner and Lloyd 1995). Parental loss in early life is also significantly over represented in the childhood histories of many who go onto be diagnosed with psychotic disorders later in adult life (Read et al. 2004), and such loss may have been the experience of many children growing up in the shadow of Indonesian occupation, exacerbated where extended family networks were dissipated, worn down or destroyed.

In this context, infant observation researchers and theorists have begun to ask questions about the *ontogeny of the self*—that is how infants and children learn to identify, reflect upon, and regulate their emotions, and distinguish between internal and external reality, however culturally configured? Parental sensitivity and attunement, *contingent* on the infants behaviour and involving a particular quality of exaggerated *mirroring* of voice, gesture and facial expression (termed *marking*) of the infants signals and emotions is theorised as enabling the infant to become aware of what emotions belong to the self, and what to the mother/caregiver, and has been consistently observed within the Western ideal of securely attached maternal-infant dyads (Fonagy et al. 2002; Gergely and Watson 1999; Holmes 2001).

While clearly demanding further research among non-Western persons, the idea that an infant becomes to know self through what is reflected back from carers, does have intuitive cross-cultural appeal. If a parent appears fearful with the infant, clearly the infant may themselves become afraid, but moreover if *marking* of the infants states is insufficiently differentiated from the carers own states, the infant is theorised as potentially construing him/herself as the source of his carer's fear. Similarly if the caregiver's responses to the infant are not really contingent and resonant with the infants own mental state, then there is a distortion of mirroring, and the infant may take in (or introject) a sense of themselves not reflective of their true nature.[18] Fonagy (2002) and colleagues have termed this the "alien self" and as such it may be disavowed and externalised, and as such provides a further productive model for the relational genesis of hallucinations. Furthermore, if multiple contradictory representations of the self, are reflected back to the infant at different times (perhaps because of changing circumstances impacting on the carers own capacities), this might be a basis for a potential failure in integration of self-concept, expressed in disorganised attachment behaviour, and its later mental corollary, dissociative states of mind.[19]

In light of this evidence concerning the importance of early experience it appears therefore significant that 4/9 of the BRR cohort documented in this study would have been infants born at the time of the initial Indonesian occupation or in the early years of the resistance, particularly as the brunt of loss and adversity in the conflict is understood to have been born in the first five years of occupation (Aditjondro 2000). An additional 3/9 would have been age 10–16, and only 2/9 would have been over the age of 18. A developmental hypothesis would predict that the earlier the family trauma the more likely the development of self is to be compromised and it is therefore of interest that there appears to be a tentative correlation (see Fig. 3.1) between age and *acute* functional impairment (note *lower scores = greater impairment*—blue line) that is not explained by lifetime trauma-event differences (red line), although of course other sociocultural factors affecting young adults are not accounted for here (see Chap. 4), and older persons may have learnt to adapt and live with intrusive symptoms to a greater extent.

How though to reconcile this observation with the almost complete inter-episodic functional recovery described for this cohort? One possible solution is the idea that a very brittle sense of self (or in psychoanalytic terms, rigid ego) might develop in as a semi-adaptive solution to earlier life deprivation or trauma (Scharfetter 2008). Scharfetter (2008, Sect. 4.6.2) likens this brittle self to "glass" which may "shatter" easily in response to further stress—whether this be further trauma, family or economic stress, illness or intoxication—leading to the loss of all coherence and manifesting in psychotic states of mind (see also Sect. 2.2.1). However equally (like molten glass) it may be capable of re-grouping, once the further stress has resolved and the *warmth* of attachment safety restored. Other dissociative conditions, including dissociative identity disorder and the dissociative subtype of PTSD, may result in a lesser degree of fragmentation, more like

[18] Such a statement may raise significant objections from those who have a strong social constructionist or narrative view of the self. It is however compatible with Hacking's (1999) idea of "interactive [human] kinds," in which nature and culture are viewed in a dialectical movement, and in which we have rooted our epistemology (see Sect. 1.7.2).

[19] We need to acknowledge much of this work and theorising derives from Western mother-child dyads, and its applications to possible extended networks of care needs further working out (cf. Howes and Spieker 2008). In an extended network it would seem unlikely that all carers would be consistent in their mirroring of the infant-child. Is this mitigated by the dominant effect of a primary caregiver, or does this inconsistency itself contribute to the higher prevalence of dissociative phenomena (not necessarily pathological) in non-Western settings and how does this contrast with the role of working mothers and professional, non-familial childcare in the West?

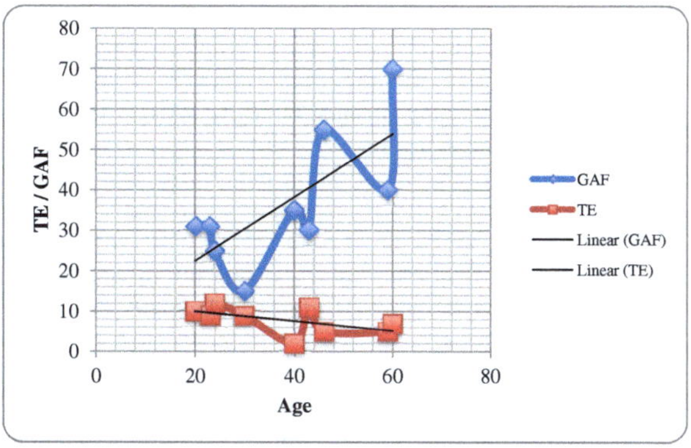

Fig. 3.1 Relationship between Age and Functional Impairment (GAF)/Lifetime Trauma Exposure (TE)

"quicksilver" organising into "little wholes" (Scharfetter 2008, Sect. 4.6.2) and we will further develop our argument in Chaps. 4 and 5 that sociocultural processes may have an organising function, delimiting fragmentation (in both time and space) and that even psychotic-like behaviour, may be more organised than initially apparent (for summary diagram see Sect. 5.3—Fig. 5.1).

References

Aditjondro, George J. 2000. Ninjas, Nanggalas, Monuments and Mossad Manuals: An anthropology of Indonesian State terror in East Timor. In *Death squad: the anthropology of state terror*, ed. Jeffrey A. Sluka, 158–88. University of Pennsylvania Press.

Ahbel-Rappe, Karin. 2006. "I no longer believe": Did freud abandon the seduction theory? *Journal of the American Psychoanalytic Association* 54(1): 171–199.

'Annotated Bibliography of Child and Forced Labor Information.' 2009. Volume II: East Timor—Kyrgyzstan. www.dol.gov/ilab/media/reports/external/Annotated_Bib_VolumeII.pdf.

Bacon, Thomas, and Angela Kennedy. 2014. Clinical perspectives on the relationship between psychosis and dissociation: Utility of structural dissociation and implications for practice. *Psychosis*, May, 1–11. doi:10.1080/17522439.2014.910252.

Becker-Blease, K.A., K. Deater-Deckard, T. Eley, J.J. Freyd, J. Stevenson, and R. Plomin. 2004. A genetic analysis of individual differences in dissociative behaviors in childhood and adolescence. *Journal of Child Psychology and Psychiatry* 45(3): 522–532.

Belsky, J., C. Jonassaint, M. Pluess, M. Stanton, B. Brummett, and R. Williams. 2009. Vulnerability genes or plasticity genes. *Molecular Psychiatry* 14(8): 746–754.

Benoit, Diane, and Kevin C.H. Parker. 1994. Stability and transmission of attachment across three generations. *Child Development* 65(5): 1444–1456. doi:10.1111/j.1467-8624.1994.tb00828.x.

Bhugra, Dinesh, and Kamaldeep Bhui. 2002. Is the Oedipal complex universal? Problems for sexual and relationship psychotherapy across cultures. *Sexual and Relationship Therapy* 17(1): 69–86. doi:10.1080/14681990220107992.

Bion, W. R. 1959. "Attacks on Linking." *International Journal of Psycho-Analysis* 40: 308−315.

Bovensiepen, Judith. 2011. Opening and closing the land: Land and power in the Idaté highlands. In *Land and life in Timor-Leste: Ethnographic essays*, ed. Andrew McWilliam, and Elizabeth G. Traube, 68–86. Canberra, ACT, Australia: ANU E Press. EPUB file.

Bracken, Pat, Philip Thomas, Sami Timimi, Eia Asen, Graham Behr, Carl Beuster, Seth Bhunnoo, et al. 2012. Psychiatry beyond the current paradigm. *The British Journal of Psychiatry* 201(6): 430–434. doi:10.1192/bjp.bp.112.109447.
Casher, Michael I., and Joshua D. Bess. 2010. *Manual of inpatient psychiatry*. Cambridge: Cambridge University Press.
Cashford, J. 2003. *The moon: Myth and image*. Basic Books.
Castagnini, Augusto C. 2010. Wimmer's concept of psychogenic psychosis revisited. *History of Psychiatry* 21(1): 54–66. doi:10.1177/0957154X09338086.
Castillo, Richard J. 1994. Spirit possession in South Asia, dissociation or hysteria? Part 1: Theoretical background. *Culture, Medicine and Psychiatry* 18(1): 1–21. doi:10.1007/BF01384875.
Cloitre, M., B.C. Stolbach, J.L. Herman, B. van der Kolk, R. Pynoos, J. Wang, and E. Petkova. 2009. A developmental approach to complex PTSD: Childhood and adult cumulative trauma as predictors of symptom complexity. *Journal of Traumatic Stress* 22(5): 399–408.
Dennett, Daniel Clement. 1993. *Consciousness explained*. London: Penguin.
Dorahy, Martin J., and Melissa J. Green. 2008. Cognitive perspectives on dissociation and psychosis: Differences in the processing of threat?' In *Psychosis, trauma and dissociation: Emerging perspectives on severe psychopathology*, eds. Andrew Moskowitz, Ingo Schäfer, and Martin Justin Dorahy, 5850–6379. Chichester, West Sussex. UK: Wiley-Blackwell. Kindle file.
Dow, J. 1986. Universal aspects of symbolic healing: A theoretical synthesis. *American Anthropologist* 88(1): 56–69.
Eigen, Michael. 2004. *The Psychotic Core*. London: Karnac Books.
Faergeman, Poul M. 1963. *Psychogenic psychoses. A description and follow-up of psychoses following psychological stress*, 1st ed. London: Butterworths.
Finkelhor, David, and Jill Korbin. 1988. Child abuse as an international issue. *Child Abuse and Neglect* 12(1): 3–23. doi:10.1016/0145-2134(88)90003-8.
Fonagy, Peter. 2001. *Attachment theory and psychoanalysis*. New York: Other Press.
Fonagy, Peter, Gyorgy Gergely, Elliot Jurist, and Mary Target. 2002. *Affect regulation, mentalization, and the development of the self*. New York: Other Press.
Freud, Sigmund. 2001a. Constructions in analysis. In *The standard edition of the complete psychological works of sigmund freud* (trans: James Strachey, Paperback, 23:255–69). London: Vintage. (Original work published 1939).
Freud, Sigmund. 2001b. Lecture XVIII: Fixations to Traumas—the Unconscious. In *The standard edition of the complete psychological works of sigmund freud* (trans: James Strachey, Paperback, 15—introductory lectures on psycho-analysis 273–85). London: Vintage. (Original work published 1917).
Gaines, Atwood D. 1991. Cultural constructivism: Sickness histories and the understanding of ethnomedicines beyond critical medical anthropologies. In *Anthropologies of medicine*, eds. Beatrix Pfleiderer and Gilles Bibeau, 221–58. Vieweg+Teubner Verlag. http://link.springer.com/chapter/10.1007/978-3-322-87859-5_17.
Gaines, Atwood D. 1992. From DSM-I to III-R; Voices of self, mastery and the other: A cultural constructivist reading of U.S. psychiatric classification. *Social Science & Medicine (1982)* 35 (1): 3–24.
Gergely, György, and John S. Watson. 1999. Early socio-emotional development: Contingency perception and the social-biofeedback model. In *Early Social Cognition: Understanding Others in the First Months of Life*, ed. Philippe Rochat, 600:101–136. Hillsdale, NJ: Lawrence Erlbaum Associates.
Gilman, Sander L. 1984. The assault on truth. freud's suppression of the seduction theory. *Medical History* 28(4): 443–444.
Griffin, M.G., P.A. Resick, and M.B. Mechanic. 1997. Objective assessment of peritraumatic dissociation: Psychophysiological indicators. *The American Journal of Psychiatry* 154(8): 1081–1088.
Hacking, Ian. 1999. *The social construction of what?* Harvard University Press.

Hamilton, Claire E. 2000. Continuity and discontinuity of attachment from infancy through adolescence. *Child Development* 71(3): 690–694.

Harrison, S. 2004. Emotional climates: Ritual, seasonality and affective disorders. *Journal of the Royal Anthropological Institute* 10(3): 583–603.

Hesse, Erik, and Mary Main. 2000. Disorganized infant, child, and adult attachment: Collapse in behavioral and attentional strategies. *Journal of the American Psychoanalytic Association* 48 (4): 1097–1127. doi:10.1177/00030651000480041101.

Hicks, David. 1984. *A maternal religion: The role of women in tetum myth and ritual*. Monograph series of Southeast Asia. Northern Illinois University, Center for Southeast Asian Studies.

Hirsch, Steven J., and Marc H. Hollender. 1969. Hysterical psychosis: clarification of the concept. *American Journal of Psychiatry* 125(7): 909–915.

Hoerl, Christoph. 2013. Jaspers on explaining and understanding in psychiatry. In *One hundred years of Karl Jaspers' general psychopathology*, eds. Thomas Fuchs and Giovanni Stanghellini, 107–20. Oxford University Press.

Hollan, Douglas. 2012. On the varieties and particularities of cultural experience. *Ethos* 40(1): 37–53. doi:10.1111/j.1548-1352.2011.01230.x.

Holmes, Jeremy. 2001. *The search for the secure base: Attachment theory and psychotherapy*. Hove, East Sussex: Psychology Press.

Hopper, Kim. 2008. Outcomes elsewhere: Course of psychosis in "other cultures". In *Society and psychosis*, eds. Craig Morgan, Kwame McKenzie, and Paul Fearon, 198–216. Cambridge University Press.

Hoshmand, Lisa Tsoi. 2007. Cultural-ecological perspectives on the understanding and assessment of trauma. In *Cross-cultural assessment of psychological trauma and PTSD*, eds. John P. Wilson and Catherine So-kum Tang, 31–50. International and cultural psychology series, Part 2. Boston, MA: Springer US.

Howell, Elizabeth F. 2014. Ferenczi's concept of identification with the aggressor: Understanding dissociative structure with interacting victim and abuser self-states. *American Journal of Psychoanalysis* 74(1): 48–59. doi:10.1057/ajp.2013.40.

Howes, Carollee, and George Spieker. 2008. Attachment relationships in the context of multiple caregivers. In *Handbook of attachment*, eds. Jude Cassidy and Phillip R. Shaver, 2nd ed., 317–332. New York, NY: Guilford Press.

Humpston, C.S. 2014. Perplexity and meaning: Toward a phenomenological "core" of psychotic experiences. *Schizophrenia Bulletin* 40(2): 240–243. doi:10.1093/schbul/sbt074.

Isaacs, Susan. 1948. The nature and function of phantasy. *The International Journal of Psychoanalysis*. http://psycnet.apa.org/psycinfo/1949-05299-001.

Jackson, Stanley W. 1986. *Melancholia and depression: From hippocratic times to modern times*. New Haven, CT: Yale University Press.

Jackson, Murray, and Paul Williams. 1994. *Unimaginable storms: A search for meaning in psychosis*. Karnac Books.

Jenkins, Janis Hunter, and Robert J. Barrett (eds.). 2004. *Schizophrenia, culture, and subjectivity: The edge of experience*. Cambridge, UK: Cambridge University Press.

Jilek, W.G., and L. Jilek-Aall. 1970. Transient psychoses in Africans. *Psychopathology* 3(6): 337–364.

Johnson, Allen W., and Douglass Richard Price-Williams. 1996. *Oedipus ubiquitous: The family complex in world folk literature*. Stanford University Press.

Jung, C. G. 1977. *Mysterium coniunctionis*. 2nd ed. vol. 14. Bollingen.

Keller, H. 2012. Attachment and culture. *Journal of Cross-Cultural Psychology* 44(2): 175–194. doi:10.1177/0022022112472253.

Kihlstrom, J.F. 1987. The cognitive unconscious. *Science* 237(4821): 1445–1452. doi:10.1126/science.3629249.

Kihlstrom, John F. 2005. Dissociative disorders. *Annual Review of Clinical Psychology* 1(1): 227–253. doi:10.1146/annurev.clinpsy.1.102803.143925.

Kirmayer, Laurence J. 1993. Healing and the invention of metaphor: The effectiveness of symbols revisited. *Culture, Medicine and Psychiatry* 17(2): 161–195. doi:10.1007/BF01379325.

Kirmayer, Laurence J. 2011. Defining and delimiting trauma-related dissociation: A view from cultural psychiatry. *Journal of Trauma & Dissociation* 12(4): 465–468. doi:10.1080/15299732.2011.570235.
Kirmayer, Laurence J. 1994. Pacing the void: Social and cultural dimensions of dissociation. In *Dissociation: Culture, mind, and body*, ed. David Spiegel, 91–122.
Kirmayer, Laurence J., and Ellen Corin. 1998. Inside knowledge: Cultural constructions of insight in psychosis. In *Insight and psychosis*, eds. Xavier Francisco Amador and Anthony S. David, 193–220. New Yotk: Oxford University Press.
Kitwood, Tom, and Kathleen Bredin. 1992. Towards a theory of dementia care: Personhood and well-being. *Ageing and Society* 12(03): 269. doi:10.1017/S0144686X0000502X.
Korbin, Jill E. 1991. Cross-cultural perspectives and research directions for the 21st century. *Child Abuse and Neglect: The International Journal* 15: 77.
Kunin, Seth Daniel. 2003. *Religion: The modern theories*. Edinburgh University Press. EPUB file.
Lakoff, George, and Mark Johnson. 2003. *Metaphors we live by*. University of Chicago Press.
Lambek, Michael. 2003. Fantasy in practice: Projection and introjection, or the witch and the spirit medium. In *Beyond rationalism: Rethinking magic, witchcraft, and sorcery*, ed. Bruce Kapferer, 198–214. Berghahn Books.
Lanius, Ruth A., Eric Vermetten, Richard J. Loewenstein, Bethany Brand, J. Christian Schmahl, Douglas Bremner, and David Spiegel. 2010. Emotion modulation in PTSD: Clinical and neurobiological evidence for a dissociative subtype. *American Journal of Psychiatry* 167(6): 640–647. doi:10.1176/appi.ajp.2009.09081168.
Lewis-Fernández, Roberto, Alfonso Martínez-Taboas, Vedat Sar, Sapana Patel, and Adeline Boatin. 2007. The cross-cultural assessment of dissociation. In *Cross-cultural assessment of psychological trauma and PTSD*, eds. John P. Wilson and Catherine So-kum Tang, 279–317. International and Cultural Psychology Series. Springer. http://link.springer.com/chapter/10.1007/978-0-387-70990-1_12.
Liotti, G. 2006. A model of dissociation based on attachment theory and research. *Journal of Trauma & Dissociation* 7(4): 55–73.
Liotti, Giovanni, and Andrew Gumley. 2008. An attachment perspective on schizophrenia: The role of disorganized attachment, dissociation and mentalization. In *Psychosis, trauma and dissociation: Emerging perspectives on severe psychopathology*, eds. Andrew Moskowitz, Ingo Schäfer, and Martin Justin Dorahy, 3769–4287. Chichester, West Sussex UK: Wiley-Blackwell. Kindle file.
Lucas, Richard. 2008. The psychotic wavelength* †. *Psychoanalytic Psychotherapy* 22(1): 54–63. doi:10.1080/02668730801962763.
Martindale, Brian, and Alison Summers. 2013. The psychodynamics of psychosis. *Advances in Psychiatric Treatment* 19(2): 124–131. doi:10.1192/apt.bp.111.009126.
Masson, Jeffrey Moussaieff. 2003. *The assault on truth: Freud's suppression of the seduction theory*. Ballantine Books.
McCrae, Niall. 2011. *The moon and madness*. Andrews UK Limited. EPUB file.
Mitchell, Stephen A., and Lewis Ed Aron, eds. 1999. *Relational psychoanalysis: The emergence of a tradition*. Vol. 14. Relational Perspectives Book Series. Analytic Press. http://psycnet.apa.org/psycinfo/1999-02491-000.
Mizen, Richard, and Mark Morris. 2006. *On aggression and violence: An analytic perspective*. Houndmills, Basingstoke, Hampshire ; New York: Palgrave Macmillan.
Moskowitz, Andrew. 2004. "Scared stiff": Catatonia as an evolutionary-based fear response. *Psychological Review* 111(4): 984.
Moskowitz, Andrew. 2008. Association and dissociation in the historical concept of schizophrenia. In *Psychosis, trauma and dissociation: Emerging perspectives on severe psychopathology*, eds Andrew Moskowitz, Ingo Schäfer, and Martin Justin Dorahy, 1475–1903. Chichester, West Sussex. UK: Wiley-Blackwell. Kindle file.
Obeyesekere. 1984. *Medusa's hair: An essay on personal symbols and religious experience*. Chicago and London: University of Chicago Press. Kindle file.

Obeyesekere, Gananath. 1990. *The work of culture: Symbolic transformation in psychoanalysis and anthropology*. University of Chicago Press.
Ortner, Sherry B. 1973. On key symbols. *American Anthropologist, New Series* 75(5): 1338–1346. doi:10.2307/674036.
Ostow, Mortimer. 1995. *Ultimate intimacy: The psychodynamics of jewish mysticism*. Karnac Books.
Parsons, Anne. 2010. Is the Oedipus complex universal? In *Psychological anthropology: A reader on self in culture*, ed. Robert A. LeVine, 131–53. John Wiley & Sons. (Original work published 1964).
Pearce, W.Barnett. 2007. *Making social worlds: A communication perspective*. Oxford, UK: Blackwell.
Pestalozzi, Julia. 2003. The symbolic and concrete: Psychotic adolescents in psychoanalytic psychotherapy. *The International Journal of Psychoanalysis* 84(3): 733–753. doi:10.1516/G6AC-WEHN-EBWM-5VD9.
Pierre Bourdieu. 1992. *The logic of practice*. (trans: Richard Nice). Stanford, California: Stanford University Press.
Read, John, Lisa Goodman, Anthony P. Morrison, Colin A. Ross, and Volkmar Aderhold. 2004. Childhood trauma, loss and stress. In *Models of madness: psychological, social and biological approaches to schizophrenia*, eds. John Read, Richard Bentall, and Loren Mosher, 223–252. Routledge.
Read, J., J. Os, A.P. Morrison, and C.A. Ross. 2005. Childhood trauma, psychosis and schizophrenia: A literature review with theoretical and clinical implications. *Acta Psychiatrica Scandinavica* 112(5): 330–350.
Reis, R. 2013. Children enacting idioms of witchcraft and spirit possession as a response to trauma: Therapeutically beneficial, and for whom? *Transcultural Psychiatry* 50(5): 622–643. doi:10.1177/1363461513503880.
Rees, S., Silove, D., Verdial, T., Tam, N., Savio, E., Fonseca, Z., Thorpe, R., et al. 2013. Intermittent explosive disorder amongst women in conflict affected Timor-Leste: associations with human rights trauma, ongoing violence, poverty, and injustice. *PLoS ONE* 8(8): e69207. doi:10.1371/journal.pone.0069207.
Ross, Colin A. 2008. Dissociative schizophrenia. In *Psychosis, trauma and dissociation: Emerging perspectives on severe psychopathology*, eds. Andrew Moskowitz, Ingo Schäfer, and Martin Justin Dorahy, 8433–8801. Chichester, West Sussex. UK: Wiley-Blackwell. Kindle file.
Sabat, Steven R. 2006. Mind, meaning, and personhood in dementia: The effects of positioning. In *Dementia: mind, meaning, and the person*, eds. Julian C. Hughes, Stephen J. Louw, and Steven R. Sabat. Oxford University Press.
Sass, Louis A. 1992. *Madness and modernism: Insanity in the light of modern art, literature, and thought*. New York, NY.: Basic Books.
Scharfetter, Christian. 2008. Ego-fragmentation in schizophrenia: A severe dissociation of self-experience. In *Psychosis, trauma and dissociation: emerging perspectives on severe psychopathology*, eds. Andrew Moskowitz, Ingo Schäfer, and Martin Justin Dorahy, 1925–2270. Chichester, West Sussex. UK: Wiley-Blackwell. Kindle file.
Seikkula, J., B. Alakare, and J. Aaltonen. 2011. The comprehensive open-dialogue approach in Western Lapland: II. Long-term stability of acute psychosis outcomes in advanced community care. *Psychosis* 3(3): 192–204.
Seligman, Rebecca, and Laurence J. Kirmayer. 2008. Dissociative experience and cultural neuroscience: Narrative, metaphor and mechanism. *Culture, Medicine and Psychiatry* 32(1): 31–64.
Shaw, D.S., and J.I. Vondra. 1993. Chronic family adversity and infant attachment security. *Journal of Child Psychology and Psychiatry* 34(7): 1205–1215.
Silove, Derrick, Robert Brooks, Catherine Robina Bateman Steel, Zachary Steel, Kalhari Hewage, James Rodger, and Ian Soosay. 2009. Explosive anger as a response to human rights violations in post-conflict Timor-Leste. *Social Science and Medicine* 69(5): 670–677. doi:10.1016/j.socscimed.2009.06.030.

da Silva, F.V. 2008. *Archeology of Intangible Heritage*. New York: Peter Lang.
Spauwen, Janneke, Lydia Krabbendam, Roselind Lieb, Hans-Ulrich Wittchen, and Jim van Os. 2006. Impact of psychological trauma on the development of psychotic symptoms: Relationship with psychosis proneness. *The British Journal of Psychiatry: The Journal of Mental Science* 188: 527–533. doi:10.1192/bjp.bp.105.011346.
Spillius, Elizabeth Bott, Jane Milton, Penelope Garvey, Cyril Couve, and Deborah Steiner. 2011. *The new dictionary of Kleinian thought*. London and New York: Routledge. Kindle file.
Summerfield, D. 2001. The invention of post-traumatic stress disorder and the social usefulness of a psychiatric category. *BMJ* 322(7278): 95–98. doi:10.1136/bmj.322.7278.95.
Tang, K. 2002. An investigation on child abuse and commercial sexual exploitation of children (csec) in East Timor. UNICEF. http://www.unicef.org/evaldatabase/index_31155.html.
Taussig, M.T. 1980. Reification and the consciousness of the patient. *Social Science & Medicine. Part B Medical Anthropology* 14(1): 3–13.
Thomas, Philip, Patrick Bracken, and Ivan Leudar. 2004. Hearing voices: A phenomenological-hermeneutic approach. *Cognitive Neuropsychiatry* 9(1–2): 13–23. doi:10.1080/13546800344000138.
Toome, Emily. 2012. "Filling wounds with salt": The pathologisation of trauma in Timor-Leste. In *Local-Global*, ed. Damian Grenfell Traversing customary community and modern nation-formation in Timor-Leste, 11: 24–30.
Traube, Elizabeth G. 1986. *Cosmology and social life: Ritual exchange among the Mambai of East Timor*. University of Chicago Press.
Turner, Victor. 1967. *The forest of symbols*. London: Cornell University Press.
Turner, R. Jay, and Donald A. Lloyd. 1995. Lifetime traumas and mental health: The significance of cumulative adversity. *Journal of Health and Social Behavior* 36(4): 360–376. doi:10.2307/2137325.
Vallée, Manuel. 2011. 'Resisting American Psychiatry: French opposition to DSM-III, biological reductionism, and the pharmaceutical ethos. In *Sociology of Diagnosis*, eds. P.J. McGann and David J. Hutson. *Advances in Medical Sociology* 12: 85–110.
van der Hart, Onno, Ellert Nijenhuis, Kathy Steele, and Daniel Brown. 2004. Trauma-related dissociation: Conceptual clarity lost and found. *Australian and New Zealand Journal of Psychiatry* 38(11–12): 906–914. doi:10.1111/j.1440-1614.2004.01480.x.
van der Hart, Onno, and Eliezer Wiztum. 2008. Dissociative psychosis: Clinical and theoretical aspects. In *Psychosis, trauma and dissociation: Emerging perspectives on severe psychopathology*, eds. Andrew Moskowitz, Ingo Schäfer, and Martin Justin Dorahy, 7759–8118. Chichester, West Sussex. UK: Wiley-Blackwell. Kindle file.
van IJzendoorn, Marinus H., and Abraham Sagi-Schwartz. 2008. Cross-cultural patterns of attachment: Universal and contextual dimensions. In *Handbook of attachment*, eds. Jude Cassidy and Phillip R. Shaver, 2nd ed., 880–905. New York, NY: Guilford Press.
West, Marcus. 2007. *Feeling, being, and the sense of self: A new perspective on identity, affect, and narcissistic disorders*. Karnac Books.
Wilson, M. 1993. DSM-III and the transformation of american psychiatry: A history. *The American Journal of Psychiatry* 150(3): 399–410.
Wimmer, August. 2003. *Psychogenic psychoses* (trans: Johan Schioldann.). Adelaide, S. Australia.: Adelaide Academic Press. (Original work published 1916).
Wiztum, Eliezer, and Onno van der Hart. 2008. Hysterical psychosis: A historical reivew and empirical overview. In *Psychosis, trauma and dissociation: Emerging perspectives on severe psychopathology*, eds. Andrew Moskowitz, Ingo Schäfer, and Martin Justin Dorahy, 1095–1457. Chichester, West Sussex. UK: Wiley-Blackwell. Kindle file.

Chapter 4
Narrative Dimensions of Dissociative-Psychosis

4.1 Narrative Violation

4.1.1 Narrative Understandings of Trauma

Complementary to the structural, psychoanalytical and relational psychological models of dissociation described in Chaps. 2 and 3, is a narrative understanding of trauma and dissociation. As Kirmayer (1996, p. 151) points out: "Trauma creates a broken narrative…in which the logic and continuity of one's life is ruptured and the story falters" such that "the very failure or impossibility of the effort to forge a coherent story makes certain events doubly traumatic." Indeed it is this failure to forge a coherent story which is also implicated in dissociative experience (Kirmayer 1994).

Many individual narratives may also be understood in relation to wider social narratives. For example the widely held social narrative of Timor-Leste's suffering that emerged through our interview process, indicated that most people felt the human cost, and subsequent economic hardship, was worth the price of achieving the reward of national sovereignty and autonomy. Writing from the Western clinical tradition, but invoking narrative implications of attachment theory (see Sect. 3.2), Holmes (1999, 59) describes dissociated/disorganised states of mind as needing a "narrative strong enough to contain traumatic pain". Within the narrative model, the evident ability of many Timorese "victims" to find such storied meaning in the face of trauma and suffering, might be argued to limit the risk of dissociative phenomenology, as the individual-group narrative is not violated beyond repair and painful affects may be tolerated and held within this higher order of meaning. Such narratives are not necessarily universally shared however, and those who do not share the sentiments behind such stories, would be predicted to be at greater risk of dissociative distress, as was borne out in interviews with many individuals experiencing high levels of mental distress, and illustrated in the case history below: a

J. Rodger and Z. Steel, *Between Trauma and the Sacred*,
Cultural Studies of Science and Medicine, DOI 10.1007/978-3-319-24424-2_4

non-psychotic middle-aged man meeting DSM-IV criteria for severe PTSD, drawn from our wider research cohort:

Rodrigo, a 35 year old, lived with his wife and children. During the independence struggle he had provided logistical support to pro-independence freedom fighters, and belonged to a clandestine pro-independence organisation. Because of this he was targeted by the Indonesian military, being subject to several beatings, one of which left him significantly injured. He admitted he lived in fear of his life. Since independence, he had been unable to find work, and relied on his family members in the countryside to provide food, which was a considerable worry for him. He felt angry about his situation and aggrieved by the lack of government recognition for those who took part in the independence struggle, particularly since he believed, with others, that many ex-militia members reportedly had managed to get better jobs, for example in the military and police, than those who had supported Independence.

Rodrigo, to some extent, presents with a coherent story (albeit a painful one) although clearly for a diagnosis of PTSD, some aspects of his suffering have not found meaningful or emotional resolution, no doubt further inflamed by economic and material insecurity, and perceived injustice. Since *narrative is essentially the "device" upon which emotion, meaning and lived experience converge in the creation and maintenance of different selves,* poverty and insecurity can themselves be partly understood as becoming subsumed within this model and his story. Where dissociative–psychotic experience arises, narrative breakdown (as both cause and consequence) is clearly more pronounced (Linington 2010; Liotti and Gumley 2008).

Indeed within the Mambai ethnolinguistic group, from which two of the BRR psychotic subjects were drawn, the story of the independence struggle and people's subsequent expectations of its personal material and economic implications, have been woven into a revised mythic narrative, highlighting a strongly held cultural code of social reciprocity, and reaching back in its claims for justice to the mythic past (Traube 2007). Summarising Traube (2007; based on pre- and post-Independence fieldwork)—the Mambai see themselves as they original autochthonous people of Timor, with primacy over even other indigenous groups. One of their myths, which has some historical basis, tells the story of a Christ-like martyred Timorese saint, called Tat Felis, who had been key in facilitating the coming of Christianity to Timor. Through this story, the whole war of independence, was seen as having been contrived to exact the ritual sacrifice of blood owed Tat Felis' for his wrongful execution in lieu of his killer's failure to complete an appropriate mortuary rite at the time. The myth further articulates emotive tensions between various Mambai groups as, to who was responsible for "killing God," but found contemporary resonance in relation to accusations of pre-Independence Indonesian-collaboration by some politically powerful villages.

According to Traube (2007, 21), what is at stake:

> is a wider vision of redistributive justice that many Mambai articulated. The formula is simple: those who pursued their own selfish interests and prospered under the occupation should be made to pay, while those who suffered and sacrificed for independence should be recompensed.

Where this is seen to happen, the elevation of contemporary suffering to the status of mythic narrative, provides what Holmes (1999, 59) calls for—a "narrative strong enough to contain traumatic pain". However as articulated by Rodrigo in our interview above, Traube (2007, 21) notes:

> a mounting apprehension, however, that just the reverse was happening in the early days of nationhood. Rather than rewarding its purchasers, many people observed, the nation seemed to favour those who had been hostile or indifferent to it, such as former collaborators and returned diasporans.

Indeed it was said to us that this was a conscious government policy to foster peace and reintegration. While it is not clear to us whether the Tat Felis myth held any currency outside of the Mambai group, it seems likely that it may have, given the appropriation of one of its key characters, a young Mambai boy called Mau Bere—whose life was said to have been taken so that Tat Felis could defeat death—as a symbol of "the people" by Fretlin, the emerging victorious government of the new Independent Timor-Leste. Even if beyond the Mambai, the Tat Felis myth was not at the forefront on people's minds, Rodrigo (not Mambai himself), does appear to be articulating with the Mambai a "commonplace that the nation was won through suffering and sacrifice; it was 'purchased'…'with the blood of the people'" evoking the "cultural code of reciprocity" (Traube 2007, 10) and thereby reminding "the nation's leaders that they expect their own wages to be paid" (22).

The widespread serious civil unrest, further internal displacement, and contingent breakdown of internal security that necessitated the reintroduction of an external peace-keeping force, in 2006, following attacks and counter-attacks along tribal and regional divisions, in a climate of growing economic division and austerity (Durand 2009) may therefore have been expected to increase rates of trauma related symptomatology (including psychosis), on the basis of both Silove and Steel's (2006) model of re-emergent physical threat, but also on account of the threat to overarching narrative meaning (and its embedded assumptions of reciprocity), that may previously have been so containing. Additionally the ongoing anxiety and unhappiness caused by material insecurity might provide the conditions (or lower the threshold) for rumination and involuntary recall of previous traumatic events (see Sect. 5.3—Fig. 5.1).

While it does not follow that everyone who had these views and experience of post-independence social inequality would be troubled with greater traumatic preoccupation, in certain individuals the balance between uncontained verses sealed-off traumatic memory may be shifted towards the former, and thereby trigger a recurrence of psychotic symptoms in those already predisposed. This may be on account of an inability to integrate such memories and painful affect into a higher order narrative, such that they remain intrusive. Clinical and anthropological work with those experiencing dissociated states of mind then, has highlighted the importance of narrative and attribution, functioning either as a counter-weight—tipping the balance back towards more organised states of mind—or in other contexts, further weighting mental processes towards greater fragmentation and chronicity.

As a further ethnographic example of Holmes' (1999, 59) idea of a "strong enough story" being able to contain and integrate dissociated/disorganised states of mind, Seligman (2005), has shown how the positively connoted, socially constituted narratives of Afro-Brazilians in north-eastern Brazil—through which dissociative experiences are interpreted as spiritual experiences of potentially healing value and provide an opportunity for passage into mediumship and initiation into the local Candomblé religion—are enough to transform, stabilise and contain dissociative experiences, *even when borne out of trauma and marginalisation*. Indeed similar arguments have been made about the constructive transformation of proto- or early psychotic states in persons called to shamanism in corresponding cultural contexts (e.g. Silverman 1967) although, in contrast to the ethnographic support now available when considering dissociative phenomena, even sympathetic critics pointed to the lack of ethnographic evidence for this argument at the time (Handelman 1968; but see Sect. 5.2.2, Footnote 16).

Obeyesekere (1984, pt. 3) uses the term "myth model" to similarly speak of the overlapping significant, often mythic, cultural meaning, shared by both audience and psychotic individual, as having similar containing and therapeutic value (see Sect. 4.2.1). Seligman and Kirmayer (2008) contrast this with the situation in the West where such experiences are usually pathologised as wholly negative, leading to a failure of meaning and integration, and a prolongation and magnification of suffering, through negative feedback looping. We contend that such a model of self, grounded in narrative, can provide a further conceptual bridge, between the anthropological model and the psychological models of dissociation (Seligman and Kirmayer 2008), claimed by some traumatologists to be mutually exclusive and incompatible (Gleaves 1996; Xiao et al. 2006; see also Sect. 3.1.4)

4.1.2 Stories Lived Verse Stories Told

To further refine our narrative argument we turn to Boddy's (1988) critical feminist analysis of *jinn*-spirit possession amongst Arabic-speaking Muslim women in the Nile villages of Northern Sudan. Boddy undertook her fieldwork in the village of Hofriyat in which she contends that nearly 50 % of woman ever married (and two-thirds of those between the ages of 35 to 55), are possessed by *zar* spirits (*zairan*). *Zairan* are understood to be red-jinn—characterised as unpredictable "pleasure-seeking, capricious, ambivalent beings"—the colour red invoking "associations of blood and human fertility" (p10). It is therefore no coincidence that the numbers are negligible in unmarried women who are yet to lay claim to the prescribed feminine-ideal of cloistered home-maker and "reproducer" (p9)—a cultural ideal not dissimilar to Hicks' (1984) characterisation of Tetum-woman in Timor-Leste.

Boddy (1988, 16) describes woman's selves in this context as "culturally overdetermined"—a process that begins in childhood, not least through the painful surgical rite of *pharaonic circumcision,*[1] that "renders her marriageable; confers on her the right to bear children; and invests her with fertility" (p6—while tempering and physically limiting sexuality not in the service of this ideal). Boddy sees woman's selfhood as constituted by excess identification with this objectified model of womanhood and builds a case that because Hofriyat notions of womanhood are so rigid and restricted, any deviation from what is culturally prescribed (e.g. through infertility or marital problems) cannot be accommodated and may lead to a dissociative *solution*.

While Boddy reasonably rejects the pathognomonic assumptions and comparisons with dissociative disorders in the West,[2] at a more broader level of analysis, invoking a narrative model of self and identity, we might draw a parallel with narrative models of pathological dissociation in which the trauma is seen as representing an extreme rupture to self-experience that cannot easily be assimilated and contained by existing narrative possibilities (Kirmayer 1996).

For the Hofriyat, however, while the rite of circumcision is no doubt painful, the trauma of this does not so much violate the sense of self as to culturally inculcate and constitute it; rather it is the unavoidable and common deviation from the inflexible cultural script of womanhood, in this context typically evoked by fertility problems in otherwise well-adjusted women, that sets the stage for culturally shaped dissociative experience. In essence this is a *dissociation of self as culturally idealised and prescribed from the self as experienced*; "between what is and what ought to be" (Boddy 1988, 17); or drawing on systemic-narrative therapy literature, because the gap between *stories lived and stories told* (cf. Pearce 2007) has become unbridgeable.

Returning to Timor-Leste another case-history from the BRR psychotic cohort is illustrative of the relevance of this understanding to our work:

Case BP6

Julinha, a 43 year old widower living with extended family was identified by them as "bulak.". Her husband had been killed by the Indonesian military when they first invaded Timor-Leste in 1975, and in 1997 she tragically lost her only two children within a month of each other, from an unidentified sickness. Presenting as

[1]Involving "excision of the labia and clitoris followed by almost complete infibulation: intentional occlusion of the vulva entailing obliteration of the vaginal meatus" (Boddy 1988, 5).

[2]Boddy (1988) makes clear the woman's *solution* can only work if the possessing other remains Other. There can be no utility in framing the possessing spirit as a projection of disowned self-experience, for this would contravene the idealised pure-feminine self that is preserved through possession, and would also be felt as an attack on kin-relations, through which the self is reciprocally interlinked (see also Sect. 5.2.1). The aim therefore is not psychic-integration, as espoused by Western therapists, although there can be ongoing communication and exchange with the possessing entity (see also Sect. 5.1.2).

chronically socially withdrawn and rarely speaking directly to others, Julinha met background DSM-IV criteria for a longstanding major depressive episode, although she was able to contribute to household maintenance and her own survival through cooking and cleaning. However during the "fulan lotuk" she was subject to brief periods of acutely disturbed psychotic-like behaviour, lasting 3–4 days, during which her usual silence was punctuated by much talking, singing and laughing, usually directed at no one, and appearing partly in response to unseen stimuli.

While in terms of Western cultural understandings Julinha certainly had reason to be *depressed*—following the emotional impact of her multiple bereavements of husband and children—this was likely further compounded by the symbolic premium placed on childbirth and fertility in Timorese culture (Hicks 2004). In other words, as with the Hofriyat above, the value of women, and the construction of female selfhood, particularly in rural, more traditional communities, continues to be largely derived through their child-bearing function—as another Timorese women put it, having recovered herself from a protracted period of "depression", which had been triggered and maintained by the death of her two previous children but alleviated by the birth of her third child, *"what use is it to have breasts without children?"*

In relation to psychosis, Julinha's chronically dysphoric state, might itself be seen as a risk factor, continually weighting her towards the possible breakdown of sealed off trauma and distress, resulting in dissociative symptoms (see Sect. 5.3—Fig. 5.1). This may parallel the patterns identified amongst the Hofriyat, in that the violation (or dissociation) of a feminine narrative self as culturally prescribed, from her self as lived and experienced, may structurally place her at risk of recurrent dissociative phenomena, especially when subject to particular personal or cultural triggers, like salient personal and cultural anniversaries or the *fulan lotuk*, with which her losses have become entwined.

The following social structural and cultural factors apparent in Timor-Leste at the time of our work may also have increased the likelihood of narrative breakdown:

(a) The gap between the *social presentation* verses the *private representation* of self necessarily increased during the period of Indonesian occupation in which the difference between outer sympathies and inner sentiments could at times be a matter of life or death. Ongoing uncertainties and instability persisting into the post-conflict period, that ultimately resulted in outbreaks of inter-group violence between 2006–2008 (see Sects. 1.3 and 4.1.1; Durand 2009), may have maintained such a gap in some individuals.
(b) A narrow margin of physical survival may make a dissociative response adaptive by keeping emotional distress *walled-off* and therefore not impeding the necessary tasks of everyday living, or as Hopper (1991, 305) puts it, in traditional societies where "permanent 'sick roles' are an unaffordable luxury…therapeutic virtue may spring from subsistence necessity." This view is

also compatible with conventional concepts of *primary gain* though which distress is kept from conscious awareness.

(c) Informal sharing of fears, needs and concerns was traditionally discouraged outside formal sanctioned settings, perhaps necessitating their *splitting off* to preserve interpersonal relationships and self-integrity. While arguably adaptive in many contexts, there is evidence that social support is an important protective factor in the aftermath of traumatic experience (Boscarino 1995). While this somewhat problematically imposes a Western understanding of "trauma" and its consequences, it may be especially relevant for societies caught between traditional practices and understanding and Western acculturation, such that traditional contexts for containing and transforming distress have been eroded but not satisfactorily replaced by new psychologies and practices. Such a situation might certainly be said to characterise the more urban areas of Timor-Leste, such as the capital Dili, with potential to influence surrounding areas, encompassing the areas where our research was conducted (see Sect. 4.2.3).

4.2 Narrative Repair

4.2.1 Culture as an Organising Narrative

In Chap. 3, we alluded to the idea that fragmented selves, may be sensitive to cultural influence, in an immediate sense, and in a different way to persons who have achieved a greater sense of coherence and established, culturally validated, sense of identity. Acutely dissociated or psychotic persons may use cultural forms, as a kind of carapace, or external scaffold, as if to compensate for a lack of internalised coherence. This may involve the taking in and articulation of cultural symbolism in quite concrete ways, particularly at moments of distress and increased dissociation—as the psychoanalyst Pestalozzi (2003, 733) puts it, "Regression to concrete thinking is understood as the chance of the psychotic patient to give some meaning to reality in an unreal, delusional world and as his/her last chance to communicate at all." It is also seems likely that the psychotic experience may find more authentic expression in non-Western cultures "that have not decoded and secularized their symbols" (Obeyesekere 1984, pt. 3: Myth Models); in other words the cosmological dramas of creation, destruction and transformation, enunciated or enacted in myth and ritual, and clearly evident within East Timorese culture. Such dramas may provide apt metaphors for the dissociative–psychotic experiences of self-fragmentation (annihilation) and subsequent reclamation—even if these are not understood metaphorically, but rather experienced in more concrete terms, by the subject (see discussion of *symbolic equations*—Sect. 3.1.2).

While psychotic persons in Western contexts may also draw on religious iconography, such as identifications with Christ (who of course embodies both death/annihilation and re-birth) it seems clear that such identifications do not provide the same totalising, and socially accepted framework that would be evident in a still strongly traditional culture such as Timor-Leste. As Obeyesekere (1984, pt. 3, Endnote 3) points out, in our secularised culture "no one accepts his fantasy: it has no cultural *meaning*" [italics in original] which we would predict to significantly curtail the efficacy of any symbolic or narrative containment. While Lucas (2004) gives an example of an high-functioning survivor of schizophrenia from Australia, who through his work as an artist, has found a level of symbolic expression analogous to the birth and death symbolism of religion, such means may be out of reach, in terms of internal and external resources, of many survivors; and while no doubt appropriate to our secular culture, may also lack the same authority as traditional religious symbolism, and may not be as containing or universally understood.

Conversely, in Timor-Leste, it was widely accepted that psychotic persons, were subject to genuine and powerful *lulik* and associated forces such as *rai nain* and the *fulan lotuk*, beyond their control, which in turn influenced the social response to such behaviour. To put it a different way, invoking the idea of Raymond Firth, "non-industrial societies may be more tolerant of the symbolisations of mental illness and are more likely to engage into a successful dialogue with them" (Littlewood and Dein 2013, 400)—something we return to in Chap. 5 (see Sect. 5.2.3), in thinking about possible links between brief and chronic psychotic states.

The psyche then is subject to both synthetic and fragmentary forces, borne of both traumatic experience and internal phantasy. If the person is to survive, and more than this, attain a level of function within the wider community, synthetic forces have to at least match, if not gain ascendance over the fragmentary. This may be achieved in different ways, for example as a stable compromise, or with oscillating states of greater and lesser coherence, distributed in time, which we have begun to argue might be the case in the phenomenon of the *fulan lotuk*. The need to function within a wider community is also more critical in a country such a Timor-Leste, lacking a social welfare system, and indeed may *necessitate* a greater degree of recovery (cf. Hopper 1991).

Importantly however, *too much integration* may bring thoughts and feelings together in such a way as to be emotionally unbearable; heightening, in Janet's terms, "mental tension" (Moskowitz 2008, Sect. 3.5), beyond what feels tenable for the individual. In such instances, a degree of dissociation, may both bring emotional relief and indeed be functionally adaptive—in contrast, as Jackson and Williams (1994) note, a lessening of projective defences may actually increase confusion as contradictory self-parts are brought into contact. Yet conversely, if sustained, dissociative states are likely to be experienced as lacking sufficient emotional contact (and may be associated with functional impairment[3]) and may consequently lead to

[3]The neuroscientist Antonio Damasio, observed "that individuals whose affective capacities were impaired also experienced cognitive impairment…rationality cannot be properly distinguished from emotions" (West 2007, 92).

a drive for greater emotional connection—thereby setting up the kind of oscillation between integration and fragmentation described in the *fulan lotuk*. In an emerging post-conflict nation such as Timor-Leste, this adaptive balance, between connection with self and the wider community, and the sealing off of distress to facilitate social, domestic and occupational (or educational) functioning, is likely to be finely balanced.

Nonetheless it is important to point out that what, to an untrained Western observer, might appear as disorganised or fragmentary, may in fact be more organised than first appearances suggest (indeed as already commented upon, in the example of dissociative-conversion predicated on lay notions of psychotic behaviour—see Sect. 3.1.4). Additionally, as noted above, wider culturally influenced narratives available to the individual may at times be sufficient to prevent a radical disjuncture in the individuals self-narrative through appeal to a higher order of meaning that may allow for greater toleration of painful affect or aberrations to lived experience. However even when the individual self-narrative does appear to breakdown this need not be seen as an entirely problematic or permanent affair in non-Western cultures that endorse the possibility of states of *involuntariness* and narrative-self *multiplicity*, often through externalised attributions of agency (cf. Kirmayer 1994). Local *lulik* and associated concepts such as *rai nain* and the effects of the *fulan lotuk* were notable examples of this in Timor-Leste.

Such non-volitional action may be seen to occur outside of normal narrative time—instead being confined to a "magical realm"—that does not require integration into the stream of conventional self-consciousness (cf. Kirmayer 1994). "Illness," in this context, may be at least partially analogous to "ritual time" (ritual, of course, like illness, being intimately bound up with *lulik*) which as Traube (1986, 21) notes is, "marked off from ordinary time and has a disposition of its own." Somewhat paradoxically then, ruptures in individual narratives, may at a higher level, be subject to tacit cultural acknowledgement, and indeed ordering or scripting, for example, in relation to *how long a rupture in experience might be expected to last, what the community's response to this should be, and what might bring about re-connection*. We will return to this concept of cultural scripting, when considering different prognostic finding in relation to brief psychotic states and in relation to links between brief and chronic psychosis (see Sect. 5.2.5).

When considering the meaning of dissociative psychotic experiences it is important to recall that containing and organising cultural templates need not take the form of consciously held, coherent, narrated stories. Individual behaviour, and its relationship to the wider context, and the communities response to this, might also constitute a form of *lived narrative*, even if not verbally articulated (cf. Pearce 2007 on "stories lived" verses "stories told"). In this light it is of interest that in his pre-Independence ethnographic study of primary Tetum speaking peoples in the eastern district of Viqueque, Hicks (2004, 21–22) reflects that "ideas concerning immortality, souls, spirits, the destination of the soul of the deceased, and the origins of humanity were not constituents of anything resembling a systematic set of cosmological notions." Similarly, in her study of the mountainous Mambai people of Aileu, Traube (1986) points to only fragments of discourse ritually enunciated, which while paired to an *imagined* narrative whole, of immense symbolic and orientating value, the latter remains largely unarticulated. As previously noted, both Hicks and Traube acknowledge that the more systematised accounts of East Timorese cosmology rendered in their ethnographies, were more a reflection of their agenda as anthropologists and subsequent search for coherence. Yet Hicks (2004, 23) goes onto conclude, that the power of Tetum culture, manifest through ritual, appears to reside in the "realm of performance rather than in that of hermeneutics." Traube (1986, 16) similarly notes that primacy of the non-verbal in Mambai ritual performance, in which for example, "percussive instruments can symbolize the entirety" (see also Sect. 2.3.4)

Moving from ritual to the arguably analogous realm of illness (Littlewood and Lipsedge 1987), such observations are consistent with de Jong's and Reis' (2010, 302) conceptualisation of an idiom of distress as containing a "symbolic dimension that…employs or *enacts* language where straightforward language does not suffice or is not allowed" [emphasis added]. The enactment of such idioms may be even more likely, where both open dialogue concerning trauma, alongside its proposed linkage with *lulik* symbols are culturally proscribed. In relation to the former we have already noted a widespread reluctance to speak of trauma, or else where acknowledged it was inevitably downplayed. As an example of a similar reluctance to speak of *lulik* matters Traube's (1986, 33) describes her tenacious attempts to elicit *lulik* narratives from the Mambai, who culturally position themselves as guardians of much ritual knowledge in Timor-Leste. For a long time her questions were resisted and invariably met with: "'That is what we fear to say.'" We might conclude that verbal articulation and linguistic understanding, is not always necessary for symbolic efficacy (whether in the realm of ritual or of illness) and may be less important than performative aspects (cf. Thompson et al. 2009).

4.2.2 Cultural Scripts of Communication and Social Response

In the words of the communication theorists Watzlawick et al. (2011, 107) "all behaviour is communication, and one cannot *not* communicate" [emphasis added]. It should be clear from the foregoing discussion, that even without words, rituals are powerful socially communicative acts, that invoke a shared sense of meaning amongst participants, even if open to personal and more idiosyncratic interpretation alongside this. However the same can be said about illness, even where the underlying disease is more clearly and primarily biological in causation and manifestation, as Sontag (1988) so clearly demonstrated for cancer and tuberculosis, in her classic text *Illness As Metaphor and AIDS and Its Metaphors*. If this is true for unambiguous physical disease states,[4] it is even more so for states of psychological

[4]Ignoring, for now, theories of psychogenic contribution to physical disease causation, and while accepting the links between physical disease and socioeconomic status.

distress and "madness," in which modes of causality are more contested, although the kinds of meaning elaborated in response to such states, will be culturally influenced. Again we return to Raymond Firth's idea, paraphrased by Littlewood and Dein (2013, 400), that "non-industrial societies may be more tolerant of the symbolisations of mental illness and are more likely to engage into a successful dialogue with them" (see also Sect. 5.2.3). We might contrast this with the "malignant social psychology" (Kitwood and Bredin 1992) and "malignant social positioning" (Sabat 2006) commonly characterising the social responses to extreme states of mind in contemporary Western society,[5] in which meaning is given to such communication, by negating, infantilising and/or stigmatising.

Such communication and the social response to it, might be understood at greater or less degrees of "symbolic remove" (cf. Obeyesekere 1990). Greater degrees of symbolic remove (at least from a Western perspective) were observed in Timor-Leste for the more commonly understood claims that the cause of a subject's psychotic behaviour, was due to *lulik* or associated factors such as *rai nain* and/or the *fulan lotuk*. While such understandings were ubiquitous, in some social networks they seemed to exist alongside more direct, and less symbolic, assertions about causes of distress (cf. Graves 2003). This was clearly seen in the case of Julinha (Sect. 4.1.2—BP6) from whom verbal communication of any form was a rarity, and yet the community were in no doubt of the cause of her mental state. While the proximal cause of acute exacerbations was culturally understood as the influence of the *fulan lotuk*, the more distal cause of her overall condition (including her vulnerability to such brief psychotic states) was additionally understood, as the local elder declared, because she had "lost her mind after her husband died;" similarly, in the words of her nephew, it was because of "thinking too much about her dead husband and children" *(hanoin barak)*. Discussions of others distress was commonly limited to speculation or assertion of the causes, in language that contained an implicit, rather than explicit, emotional quality.[6]

[5]While these terms were originally framed toward a critical analysis of social and societal responses to dementia (Kitwood and Bredin 1992; Sabat 2006), they remain apt for a similar understanding of psychosis (Adams 1996).

[6]This was not necessarily, as Leff (1988) suggests in his analysis of some traditional cultures, because of a limited emotional lexicon. Tetum provided for a complex emotional range of expression, with meaning often created through the compounding of body-part words with adjoined adjectives (Avram 2008—e.g. *laran kanik* = inside broken = broken heart). As one native speaker put it to linguist Taylor-Leech (2008, 166) "I love Tetum-Terik. I am discovering more and more every day of its intricacies." Clearly however language evolves in accordance with the needs of the people using it and East Timorese ritually governed, sociocentric selves (see Sect. 1.7.2, Footnote 32) likely have less need for making subtle differentiations in internal mental states, where preferred emphasis is on relationships and meaning. Nonetheless Indonesian or Portuguese loan words could be used where necessary, particularly for technical translations of Western psychiatric terminology (such as for depression and specific psychotic symptomatology) although some may have resisted the use of loan words, especially Indonesian ones, on account of its imperialistic connotative significance (Taylor-Leech 2008).

The symbolisations of mental illness were therefore both tolerated and engaged with (see Sect. 5.2.3). Whether of greater or less symbolic remove, the cause is seen as external but *relational.* Positions of less symbolic remove bring us closer to the emergent Western understanding linking trauma, loss, adversity and psychosis (as expounded in Sects. 2.2.1 and 5.1.3). We shall go on to argue, that such externalisation may also help separate out and compartmentalise a core healthy self, from the traumatised self, in terms of managing individual experience, in addition to also serving this function relationally—by preserving the core social identity of the person, to whom others may relate, from the psychotic-part, seen as caused by trauma or *lulik* affliction—which may have an important bearing on prognosis (see Sect. 5.2.1).

To reiterate all behaviour then, whether intended or not, might be seen as communicative. Even if such meaning is bestowed by recipients, and beyond the conscious or unconscious intent of the psychotic individual, we might see particular social responses (for example, as for Julinha above) as elaborating on a rudimentary symbolism, that is ultimately constructive for the individual. To communication however we might also add a functional perspective (Jones 1993). Where fragmentation of mind is not complete, or subject to competing synthetic influences as earlier outlined, notions of primary gain, keeping full awareness of distress partially out individual experience is evident. From the perspective of a systemically informed attachment theory, symptoms might partly be viewed as different relational strategies, attempting to communicate needs and distress, and influence the kind of response engendered to these needs (Dallos and Vetere 2009). A culturally informed attachment theory (see Sect. 3.2) is able to situate such presumed universal motivations, within a cultural framework, that shapes and delimits the communicative forms available to the individual (although the individual can be seen as contesting and transforming these).

For example, in contrast to idioms of distress in the West, in his analysis of brief psychotic episodes in Swaziland, Guinness argues that suicidal gestures, or actual episodes of self-harm, far from mobilising community resources, would be instead met with contempt or "shunning" by the individuals social group, compounding the protagonists socially dislocated position (Guinness 1992).[7] In contrast more overtly "mad" or psychotic-like behaviour, similar to that observed in Timor-Leste, appear to activate an organised and purposeful social response around the individual in the throes of crisis, and thereby becomes an acceptable cultural template for appropriation in dissociative states.[8] This was certainly the case in Timor-Leste, now a deeply Catholic country, in which expression of suicidal ideation, gestures or attempts were not reported throughout the course of our study. Indeed questions

[7]While individuals in the West may be subject to the wider forces of social exclusion, acute gestures of self-harm are still recognised and responded to by the community and public service providers.

[8]Such cultural templates are part of a small repertoire of cultural resources available to the individual experiencing states of extreme mental fragmentation, functioning as an opposing "organising" influence, even if from the perspective of the observer, this is not at first apparent.

alluding to such feelings were met with surprise ("but who would look after my children"), or scorn and moral condemnation. In contrast, individuals believed to be under the spell of the *fulan lotuk* or *rai nain* were described with compassion and treated with acceptance and concern by the local community. Help would be mobilised and advice/treatment would be sought out, often involving considerable expense where traditional healers were concerned. In short their problems were seen as legitimate and taken seriously.

Idioms of dissociation, as Boddy (1994) points out, allow for expressions of distress without directly implicating or blaming others, yet clearly appear to largely locate causality outside the individual—preserving the "everyday self" from accountability and enabling normal social relations to continue at times of wellness, while enactment of the possessed self opens up new possibilities of self-experience, and associated spheres of possible action and influence, not necessarily seen as pathological, or at least of ambiguous status. For example, one of the BRR cohort, *Luciano* (Sect. 2.3.4—Table 2.1—Case BP7), *a married man in his 30s who struggled to find sufficient work, and who frequently took to drink, blames a rai nain for "making him" have sexual relations with another women in 1987 and getting her pregnant.* Whether his wife or the community fully accepted this explanation or whether he was thought to be fabricating such an explanation is uncertain[9] but he still lives with his wife and the periodic influence of the *fulan lotuk* is perhaps a reminder of his asserted limited responsibility, and perhaps also possibility of future transgression.

Social mobilisation also includes entry into the sick role—which may grant certain exemptions from everyday expectations of chores and socialisation, consistent with the concept of secondary gain seen in Western dissociative disorders. While the rules and expectation of the sick role will vary across cultures, similarities are also evident. Adriano's (Sect. 1.4.2—Case BP1) family "tread softly" around him and appear to have reduced expectations of him regarding domestic and occupational responsibility—even in between acute exacerbations. The ever-present awareness of the deleterious effects of "stressing him" and the periodicity of the *fulan lotuk* allows him ongoing community participation and negotiation under his own terms.

Previous analysis of culturally configured patterns of distress have helpfully shown that an analogous pattern analogous to ritual, of social extrusion, followed by symbolic exaggeration or inversion, and finally restitution and even social redress may be achieved through the cultural work of "illness"(Littlewood and Lipsedge 1987). More recently Wilce (2004) has argued from ethnographic work in

---

[9]According to an earlier focus group the East Timorese community acknowledged there might be occasional instances in which people simulate *bulak* with various motives (Graves 2003, 18) and indeed one participant had pertinently contented that some "people pretended to be crazy because they are drunk". At one level this in fact supports our concept of *bulak* as a culturally category to "act into" (cf. Pearce 2007; see Sect. 1.7.1). It also highlights there is likely to be a spectrum of presentations according to greater or lesser degrees of actual or apparent agency, which itself may be more or less consciously accessible.

Bangladesh that such inversions are of the sociocentric self, such that states of madness are indexed by an excess emphasis on subjectivity (and self-assertion) over more a more culturally valued intersubjectivity.

Such a model fits well with our observations in Timor-Leste and it remains productive to apply Littlewood's (2002) and Lipsedge's (Littlewood and Lipsedge 1987) ritual-illness model to many of the cases described—most, if not all of whom, occupied socially marginalized positions. For some this was often down to relative social isolation following death or displacement of family and kinsmen, for others it appeared derivative of an inability to find a meaningful role within the community. In particular this was an issue for the large number of unemployed young men, often seen roaming the streets or playing billiards, no longer able to achieve selfhood through traditional means or honour through gainful activity or resistance activities (although the many gangs of machete wielding martial arts specialists—cf. Scambary et al. 2006—may have been at some level attempting to recreate such a source of identity).

Exaggeration, but not commonly transgression, of gender stereotypes, while in the throes of acute distress, are evinced in the differential descriptions of men and women. The former were often described as "rampaging wildly through the fields" or up in the mountains, while the expression of distress in women—with the exception of Julinha (Sect. 4.1.2—Case BP6) whose gender position on account of being both widowed and bereaved of her children was arguably more ambiguous—was mostly observed or described as confined to the homestead. Such observations are comparable with ethnographic descriptions of gender-differentiated behaviour in many culture bound syndromes in different settings, including the West (Littlewood 2002)

An further analysis of Adriano's behaviour described earlier (Sect. 1.4.2—Case BP1) provides a good example of the model's hermeneutic power. Being male, unemployed, unmarried, in his late 20 s, and appearing to live in the shadow of his higher status older brother, it is perhaps not surprising that in the throes of his psychotic-like states, that this same brother became a frequent target of his attacks, including the attempted fire-setting of his brother's home. However significant injury to either party, or their audience, despite the reported brandishing of machetes, had surprisingly somehow been avoided. Indeed a similar analysis might be made for many of the transient but acutely psychotic males described in our study, in whom despite aggressive posturing and degrees of violence, serious injury was rarely described. Such a pattern is reminiscent of the *negi-negi*, or "wildman behaviour", historically described in the not so distant New Guinean Highlands, which also bears many hallmarks of dissociative behaviour here described (Littlewood and Lipsedge 1987, 291) :

> The affected man rushes about erratically, threatening people with weapons, destroying their property, blundering through the village gardens tearing up crops. Episodes last for a few hours, or at most, days; during them the wild man fails to recognize people and, on recovering, claims amnesia for the episode. Behavior is locally attributed to possession by spirits ... The incipient wild man's initial announcement that he no longer wishes to eat and his rejection of his share of the prepared food, advertize his coming performance (Clarke

1973: 209). This is always public... The audience participate by feigning terror...To observers he retains a high degree of control... In negi-negi and similar reactions there is "a disproportion between the injury threatened and actually inflicted. It is generally more alarming to the white onlooker than the native" (Seligman 1928).

This appears in stark contrast to another regionally infamous culturally-specific reaction, also bearing dissociative hallmarks, that of *amok*, which by definition ends in attempted or completed suicide or homicide or both. If we are to defend a functionalist explanation for such behaviour, how is it possible to reconcile these different culturally patterned illness manifestations? Littlewood (2002, 95–96) points out that such socially scripted models of protest would remain ineffective if injury and violence were completely unknown, or where involuntariness was doubted (see Case BP7—Luciano—above); but equally completed suicide or homicide and incarceration rules out any useful socially strategic function for the protagonist—save that of "posthumous redemption", or "retributive fantasy". Necessarily then "any instrumentality of amok lies in threat not completion" (Littlewood 2002, 95). Perhaps the scar under Adriano's eye, suggestive of at least one previous machete wound, serves as a reminder of the ever-present potential for real injury, to self or others.

We might also view the madness of Adriano, at some level, as an example of inversion—of the valued masculine role, as embodied in the evangelised powers of resistance fighters—frequently described to us in accounts by indigenous staff and those interviewed: stories in which fighters wielded *power over magic* to attack, conceal and defend themselves from their enemies. For Adriano and other afflicted men in our story it was a kind of *magic which welded power over the men* causing them to attack, not their sworn enemies but their own kinsmen.

While ideas of *scripted behaviour* remain useful[10] recent ethnographic accounts take issue with the idea of such conscious collusion between protagonist and audience, even in circumstances where the dissociative behaviour is contained within more explicit ritual structures. As a local observer of the *Toraja Maro* possession ceremony of South Sulawesi Island in North Eastern Indonesia, remarked, "'I am afraid to watch. Especially if they use knives or a machete [to apparently cut themselves]. Eeh! I am very frightened to see that!'" [parentheses in original], which when combined with other accounts leads the psychoanalytically minded anthropologist, Hollan (2000, 550) to conclude that this Maro ceremony was "in fact, rife with anxiety, for the spectators as well as for the possessed".

Even our own experience of theatre, in which we are asked more consciously to "suspend disbelief" should confirm the very real emotional, indeed cathartic, effect of such performance on the audience. Actors have testified to the power of role and enactment to evoke powerful emotion; and while there is little research in this area,

[10]A similar performance analysis has been made for dissociative experiences in Western medical settings, as manifest in the medical dramas involving patients with *conversation symptoms* taking centre stage and weaving a complex plot between patient, doctor and family, even if the "actors" are not always consciously party to the dramatic ironies, "uncovered" by later historical and cultural commentators (Ellenberger 1981; Littlewood and Lipsedge 1987).

there are case reports in both the professional and lay media, of actors who have not fully recovered (or even taken their own life) after enacting states of madness or cruelty on the stage or the screen[11] ('Are Psychotic Roles Hazardous to an Actor's Health? | PopEater.com' 2011; Igwe and Erojikwe 2014). Deeley (2003) proposes that the imaginational absorption required to get into role, using the method acting technique, is analogous to states of dissociation. Forensic psychologist, Raymond Hamden, who has given several media interviews, goes further suggesting that actors who develop such difficulties, may already be prone to dissociative tendencies, and indeed may have chosen acting as a profession, as a means to inhabit new selves, in preference to the restricted realities of their own lives (pers. comm.); a proposition not dissimilar to anthropological models of dissociation discussed (Boddy 1988, 1994). Lay commentators, have consequently pointed to the need for actors, to be well grounded in their personal lives outside off the stage, as an important factor, protecting against the development of such problems ('Are Psychotic Roles Hazardous to an Actor's Health? | PopEater.com' 2011). In the more unpredictable intrapsychic and social worlds associated with often dramatic psychotic—dissociative phenomena, the cognitive-emotional impact can only be presumed to be higher. Once again we might invoke Bourdieu's (1992, 73) aphorism: "The body believes what it plays at: it weeps if it mimes grief"—however the rest of this quote takes us full-circle, hinting at the possible unsymbolised traumatic origins to what is "mimed"—"It does not represent what it performs, it does not memorize the past, it enacts the past, brings it back to life".

In highlighting socially communicative and instrumental aspects we of course move back towards a psychoanalytic position, where needs and desires once again have a part, and behaviour may be viewed as, at least partly, unconsciously motivated. It does not reject the structural model of dissociation (especially if framed within a narrative-cultural model) but assumes that even within fractured self-subsystems, needs and drives, are still trying to assert themselves—but their task made even harder by virtue of their fragmentation. Since dissociative experience is, by definition, disorganised, and usually linked to overwhelming affect (even if this is sealed-off), it might be argued to represent, ontologically, *experience "looking" for a story or guiding narrative*—to provide organisation and meaning "strong enough to contain traumatic pain" (Holmes 1999, 59).

Local cultural templates, like that of the *fulan lotuk*, provide such a template, bringing organisation, meaning and containment, in which transients states of chaos and extreme distress are permitted and expressed through an idiom of madness, within a higher order system of meaning that simultaneously prescribes a temporal limit for such deviation and provides an expectation and structure for its tentative resolution. The ontological drive from fragmentation to coherence as negotiated through assimilation into existing or evolving cultural scripts provide a model for understanding the assumed, but undertheorised concept of *cultural pathoplasticity*,

[11]Here we might again invoke Segal's idea of "symbolic equation" (see Sect. 3.1.2), as in such instances, there is clearly a conflation between representation and reality.

as applied to dissociative states (see Sects. 1.1 and 1.5). Culture may provide potential organising narratives although this may be in the form of behavioural rather than "textual scripts" (a point, as discussed, supported by Hicks' and Traube's ethnographies in Timor-Leste).

The transient psychotic-like phenomena of the *fulan lotuk* may therefore be more organised than it appears—since complete failure of psychodynamic defences, or dissociative sealing-off is unlikely sustainable for long, and fragmentary forces are likely to exist alongside opposing synthetic ones—facilitated by the social response and cultural forms described here. We argue this may contribute to delimiting psychotic states in time and allowing some degree of adaptiveness and resilience (especially in the context of a narrow margin of survival (cf. Hopper 1991).

4.2.3 Cultural Revitalisation—Contesting Emergent Cultural Scripts

Erosion of traditional cultural beliefs and practices has been apparent in Timor-Leste, on account of at least three major forces (see also Sect. 2.3.1):

(i) Indonesian occupation and associated policies of intentional cultural violation and destruction.[12]
(ii) Syncretisation of Roman Catholic belief and practice. While Catholic missionaries were a longstanding and tolerated presence on the island from the days of the early missionaries, the Roman Catholic church did not become widely accepted until the period of Indonesian occupation, at which point it became both a symbolic and de facto bastion of resistance (Kohen 2001).
(iii) Intentional Westernisation, via the political, peace-keeping, economic, medical and educational developmental initiatives of the UN and NGOs, alongside the influential interpersonal presence of ex-pat personnel. To this we might add the "unintentional" impact of the Western presence—created through a barrage of Western imports[13] (including widespread satellite television installations—even in the many corrugated-iron rudimentary dwellings—an illicit DVD and CD market, increasing internet access and social media uptake, and widely available mobile phone technology).

[12]Another reading of Adriano's (Sect. 1.4.2—Case BP1) assertion that he "had been witness to the murder of family and/or friends"—later retracted and denied by his family—might be at the allegorical level (but experienced as concrete and real—Sects. 3.1.2 and 4.2.1) standing for his sense of wounding of Timor as a whole, although of course other explanations such as the sealing over of dissociated memory and the downplaying of trauma by his family need to be seriously considered (see Sect. 2.3.4).

[13]A neo-Marxist perspective, would of course suggest such developments to be far from incidental (even if not consciously conspiratorial) but rather part of the wider logic of late capitalist, neo-colonialism.

While many young people, including some of our own staff, acknowledged Western aspirations, both narrower and broader forces of acculturation may be consciously or unconsciously resisted, in greater or lesser measure, if felt to threaten established ways of relating and being; particularly for those who have come to feel vulnerable or distressed under the emerging new order. It is therefore prudent to look not only at mind and behaviour in the context of downward cultural forces, but also at the reciprocal effect of behaviour and inferred mental states on culture (cf. Pearce 2007). For states of mind and behaviour such as the dramatic brief-psychotic presentations, believed to be occurring under the influence of unseen *lulik* and associated forces, might in fact function—at a higher level of analysis—to re-confirm and render visible the ongoing plausibility of these hidden cultural realities. "Illness" may then yet be seen to function as a form of cultural revitalisation—not so dissimilar to the millennial or messianic cults, described so vividly in historical ethnography (e.g. Worsley 1987). Indeed the behaviour of possessed but prophetic individuals starring in the classic revitalisation movements, of such ethnography, shared many of the dissociative-like features (high drama, perceived involuntariness, and amnesia) with our own protagonists.

Perhaps unwittingly then, in addition to its more immediate effects involving the subject and his/her direct community, the afflicted subject is, more distally ensuring the enduring survival of threatened cultural forms. Significantly there exists some ethnographic evidence, and anthropological theorising, that suggests when the performance of long standing cultural rituals in a society begins to wane, a pattern of psychological distress may emerge to take its place—that symbolically can be read as attempting to articulate and resolve the same social conflicts previously addressed by the ritual in question (Littlewood 1990; see Sect. 2.3.4). Perhaps in the times of Indonesian occupation, with the threat of cultural assimilation or worse, annihilation (Aditjondro 2000), such reactions may have taken on an even greater significance (see Sect. 2.3.4).

For this reasons we must be cautious if re-framing such reactions according to a *de-contextualised* and *non-relational* Western illness model—for then, albeit also unwittingly, we ourselves de-politicise and render impotent such behaviour, making ourselves potentially complicit with earlier colonising agendas (cf. Toome 2012 on the medicalisation of trauma in Timor-Leste; cf. Ugarte 1992 in relation to amok); although this does not imply distress should be ignored.

The problem with such explanations, that we might gloss as "individual sacrifice on the altar of cultural longevity," is that an understanding of how such processes occur, or what benefit they bring to the individual (especially post Dawkins, *The Selfish Gene*) remain under-theorised. From an evolutionary perspective, the concept of sacrifice is also difficult to reconcile with individual advantage, or even in this context, with an advantage to those bearing high degrees of shared genetic inheritance (i.e. close family members; cf. Dawkins 1989). However this ignores the important healing function that an attempted, at least partial, return to a traditional cultural identity, may have (Gone 2013). Furthermore amongst contemporary evolutionary biologists, the concept of group selection has once more gained credence, operating in parallel to individual genetic selection (Wilson and Wilson

2008). In the context of our work, improved cultural cohesion and group-esteem, brought about by "individual sacrifice", might benefit all, including the afflicted individual.

We might also view this phenomena of cultural revitalisation as arising through the subjects' immersion and conjoint construction through culture, consistent with our earlier analysis of communication and illness function. Adapting Pearce's (1994, 2005) "atomic" (later re-named "daisy") dialogical-model from his group's wider *Coordinated Management of Meaning* (CMM) framework, we can see that individuals are intersubjectively constituted and therefore in continual *reciprocal dialogue* with intersubjectively constituted parts of themselves including: their *private self* (which may include psychodynamic considerations); their *public self* (as construed in different relationships, and overlapping to varying degrees with the private self); and their *idealised self* (as culturally prescribed and understand, although often confused at times of cultural change)—that all converge on a particular episode (of behaviour or speech), in interpersonal context.

This allows for an appreciation of how different pathways described in this book may recursively come together, reciprocally influencing each other, to greater or lesser degree. While within CMM's "hierarchical model" (Pearce 2005) individual acts are understood to be embedded within a hierarchical order, *usually* with higher cultural-contextual forces acting *downwards*, presumed to be stronger than individual-episodic forces acting *upwards*, it also allows for the combined power of multiple *episodes* acting upwards that could together be enough to challenge or reinforce overarching cultural meanings (Burnham and Harris 1995)—in this context to partly restore more traditional cultural positions threatened by processes of acculturation.

In the context of our work, an *episode* might be defined as the dramatic individual enactment of psychotic speech or behaviour, circumscribed in time, but which is given added salience and meaning by the impact and anticipation of its common, even cyclical lunar, recurrence. Through this process, the cultural realities of *lulik* and associated powers are repeatedly affirmed through each episode of behaviour and social response (including the seeking and intervention of traditional healers) and the subsequent re-telling in multiple contexts (including opportunities for further narrating provided for in our study). Of course it is possible with growing Westernisation that community members may increasingly come to interpret such behaviour as evidence, not of *lulik* and associated realties, but of brain disease and faulty genes[14]—yet the East Timorese have shown themselves to

[14]Indeed an earlier scoping study using community focus groups and surveys had surprisingly identified "problems with the brain" as the most frequently cited explanation for mental illness—this was contrary to our experience in the field in which this was only rarely described as an explanation (an understandable exception being the elderly lady with apparent dementia secondary to head-injury: Sects. 1.4.3 and 2.3.4—Table 2.1—Case CP4). While certainly of value, the study was linked to the setting up of the new East Timor Mental Health Service, partly funded by overseas aid, with leadership by Western mental health professionals. This scoping study was also participated in with an expectation of "psychoeducation" and as such these findings almost certainly partly reflected "demand characteristics" of the study (cf. Kagee 2004; see Sect. 1.6).

be adept at moving between registers of meaning according to context and the tenacity of important anchoring and orientating traditional beliefs was notable in all groups regardless of educational opportunity. Whatever globalisation may bring, local identities are at stake, and the visibility of psychotic behaviour provides an opportunity for all to affirm these traditionally understood veiled realities.

Implicit here again is the notion that even apparently "disorganised" psychotic states of mind, may be subject to some organisation through cultural scripts (see Sect. 5.2.5) even if it is evident that the rudimentary symbolism embedded within psychotic speech and behaviour is taken up by others, and responded to, as significant (Sects. 3.1.2, 4.2.1, 4.2.2 and 5.2.3). It has been argued by some however, that creative cultural innovation may be catalysed, in particular instances, by individuals experiencing altered mental states, including dissociation (Boddy 1994) and psychosis (Littlewood 2006), and the possibility of new emergent cultural forms, arising out of states of "illness" cannot be ruled out. Such forms may be regressive, conservative or genuinely innovative.

Timor itself remains in a state of cultural transition, caught between older traditions and more modernising Western influences, the latter linked to the foreign aid and development agenda. In this context it is perhaps significant that Adriano (Sect. 1.4.2—Case BP1) demonstrated an ironic degree of self-control in his relation to us while apparently psychotically-distressed. This was made known to us on two occasions: once while interviewing a neighbouring lady a couple of roads away from Adriano's home, in a quasi-disorganised and psychotic state, Adriano sundered onto the veranda of his neighbours home appearing hostile, yet simultaneously requesting medicine from us. His request was non-confrontationally postponed, and he was shepherded away by a neighbour's son. On another occasion he aggressively accosted us in our vehicle, to ask if we had any food we could give him. This incongruence between attitude and request perhaps represented an understandable ambivalence to our presence, representing both potential material gain (medicine, food) but also a further threat to the forms of cultural identity that were increasingly unavailable to him, and which his behaviour at one level may have been seeking to resurrect.

References

Adams, T. 1996. Kitwood's Approach to Dementia and Dementia Care: A Critical but Appreciative Review. *Journal of Advanced Nursing* 23(5): 948–953. doi:10.1046/j.1365-2648.1996.10613.x.

Aditjondro, George J. 2000. Ninjas, Nanggalas, monuments and Mossad manuals: An anthropology of Indonesian state terror in East Timor. In *Death squad: The anthropology of state terror*, ed. Jeffrey A. Sluka, 158–88. University of Pennsylvania Press.

Are Psychotic Roles Hazardous to an Actor's Health? | PopEater.com. 2011. *PopEater*. Accessed Dec 13, 2014. http://www.popeater.com/2010/12/31/disturbing-movie-roles-health-effects/.

Avram, Andrei A. 2008. An overview of reduplication and compounding in Tetun Dili. *Revue Roumaine de Linguistique* 53(4): 427–448.

Boddy, J. 1988. Spirits and selves in Northern Sudan: The cultural therapeutics of possession and trance. *American Ethnologist* 15(1): 4–27.

Boddy, J. 1994. Spirit possession revisited: Beyond instrumentality. *Annual Review of Anthropology* 23: 407–434.

Boscarino, J.A. 1995. Post-traumatic stress and associated disorders among Vietnam veterans: The significance of combat exposure and social support. *Journal of Traumatic Stress* 8(2): 317–336.

Burnham, John, and Queenie Harris. 1995. Emerging ethnicity—a tale of three cultures. In *Meeting the needs of ethnic minority children: Including refugee, black and mixed parentage children: A hanbook for professionals*, 2nd rd., eds. Kedar Nath Dwivedi and Ved P. Varma. London: Jessica Kingsley Publishers.

Dallos, Rudi, and Arlene, Vetere. 2009. *Systemic therapy and attachment narratives*. UK: Taylor & Francis.

Dawkins, Richard. 1989. *The selfish gene*. Oxford: Oxford University Press.

Deeley, Peter Q. 2003. Social, cognitive, and neural constraints on subjectivity and agency: Implications for dissociative identity disorder. *Philosophy, Psychiatry, and Psychology* 10(2): 161–167. doi:10.1353/ppp.2003.0095.

de Jong, Joop T., and Ria Reis. 2010. Kiyang-Yang, a West-African postwar idiom of distress. *Culture, Medicine and Psychiatry* 34(2): 301–321. doi:10.1007/s11013-010-9178-7.

Durand, F. 2009. Recurring crises in Timor-Leste failed state or country in search of a project? *Lusotopie* 16(2): 65–81.

Ellenberger, Henri F. 1981. *The discovery of the unconscious: The history and evolution of dynamic psychiatry*. Basic Books.

Gleaves, D.H. 1996. The sociocognitive model of dissociative identity disorder: A reexamination of the evidence. *Psychological Bulletin* 120: 42–59.

Gone, Joseph P. 2013. Redressing first nations historical Trauma: Theorizing mechanisms for indigenous culture as mental health treatment. *Transcultural Psychiatry* 50(5): 683–706. doi:10.1177/1363461513487669.

Graves, Jenni. 2003. Knowledge, attitudes and responses to mental illness. Democratic Republic of East Timor: East Timor national mental health project, Ministry of Health.

Guinness, E A. 1992. Relationship between the neuroses and brief reactive psychosis: Descriptive case studies in Africa. *The British Journal of Psychiatry. Supplement* 16: 12–23.

Handelman, Don. 1968. Shamanizing on an empty stomach. *American Anthropologist* 70(2): 353–356. New Series.

Hicks, David. 1984. *A maternal religion: The role of women in Tetum Myth and Ritual.* Monograph Series of Southeast Asia. Northern Illinois University, Center for Southeast Asian Studies.

Hicks, D. 2004. *Tetum ghosts and kin: Fertility and gender in East Timor*. 2nd edn. USA: Waveland Pr Inc.

Hollan, Douglas. 2000. Culture and dissociation in Toraja. *Transcultural Psychiatry* 37(4): 545–559. doi:10.1177/136346150003700404.

Holmes, Jeremy. 1999. Defensive and creative uses of narrative in psychotherapy: An attachment perspective. In *Healing stories: Narrative in psychiatry and psychotherapy*, eds. Glenn Roberts, and Jeremy Holmes, 49–68. Oxford, UK: Oxford University Press.

Hopper, Kim. 1991. Some old questions for the new cross-cultural psychiatry. *Medical Anthropology Quarterly* 5(4): 299–330. New Series.

Igwe, Ezinne, and Ikechukwu Erojikwe. 2014. Beyond the stage-psychosis and transport in selected performances. *Global Journal of Arts Humanities and Social Sciences* 2(9): 79–90.

Jackson, Murray, and Paul, Williams. 1994. *Unimaginable storms: A Search for meaning in psychosis*. London: Karnac Books.

Jones, Elsa. 1993. *Family Systems Therapy: Developments in the Milan-Systemic Therapies*. Wiley-Blackwell.

Kirmayer, Laurence J. 1994. Pacing the void: Social and cultural dimensions of dissociation. In *Dissociation: Culture, mind, and body*, ed. David Spiegel, 91–122.

Kirmayer, L.J. 1996. Confusion of the senses: Implications of ethnocultural variations in somatoform and dissociative disorders for PTSD. In *Ethnocultural aspects of posttraumatic stress disorder: Issues, research, and clinical applications*, eds. Anthony J. Marsella, Matthew J. Friedman, Ellen T. Gerrity, and Raymond M. Scurfield, 131–163. Washington, DC: American Psychological Association.

Kitwood, Tom, and Kathleen Bredin. 1992. Towards a theory of dementia care: Personhood and well-being. *Ageing and Society* 12(03): 269. doi:10.1017/S0144686X0000502X.

Kohen, Arnold S. 2001. The Catholic Church and the Independence of East Timor. In *Bitter flowers, sweet flowers: East Timor, Indonesia, and the world community*, eds. Richard Tanter, Mark Selden, and Stephen Rosskamm Shalom, 43–51. Lanham, Maryland: Rowman & Littlefield.

Leff, Julian. 1988. *Psychiatry around the globe: A transcultural view*. London: Gaskell.

Linington, Mark. 2010. In bits: Hearing the fragmented narratives of people who experience psychosis. In *Telling stories? Attachment based approach to the treatment of psychosis*, ed. Sarah Benamer, 113–124. London: Karnac Books.

Liotti, Giovanni, and Andrew, Gumley. 2008. An attachment perspective on schizophrenia: The role of disorganized attachment, dissociation and mentalization. In *Psychosis, trauma and dissociation: Emerging perspectives on severe psychopathology*, eds. Andrew Moskowitz, Ingo Schäfer, and Martin Justin Dorahy, 3769–4287. Chichester, West Sussex, UK: Wiley (Kindle file).

Littlewood, Roland. 1990. How universal is something we can call "Therapy"? Some implications of non-western healing systems for intercultural work. *Journal of Interprofessional Care* 5(2): 49–65. doi:10.3109/13561829009043447.

Littlewood, R. 2002. *Pathologies of the west: An anthropology of mental illness in Europe and America*. NY: Continuum International Publishing Group.

Littlewood, R. 2006. *Pathology and identity: The work of mother earth in Trinidad*. Cambridge: Cambridge University Press.

Littlewood, Roland, and Simon Dein. 2013. Did Christianity lead to schizophrenia? Psychosis, psychology and self reference. *Transcultural Psychiatry* 50(3): 397–420. doi:10.1177/1363461513489681.

Littlewood, Roland, and Maurice Lipsedge. 1987. The butterfly and the serpent: Culture, psychopathology and biomedicine. *Culture, Medicine and Psychiatry* 11(3): 289–335.

Lucas, Rod. 2004. In and out of culture: Ethnographic means to interpreting schizophrenia. In *Schizophrenia, culture, and subjectivity: The edge of experience*, eds. Janis Hunter Jenkins and Robert J. Barrett, 146–163. Cambridge, UK: Cambridge University Press.

Moskowitz, Andrew. 2008. Association and dissociation in the historical concept of schizophrenia. In *Psychosis, trauma and dissociation: Emerging perspectives on severe psychopathology*, eds. Andrew Moskowitz, Ingo Schäfer, and Martin Justin Dorahy, 1475–1903. Chichester, West Sussex, UK: Wiley-Blackwell (Kindle file).

Obeyesekere, G. 1984. *Medusa's hair: An essay on personal symbols and religious experience*. Chicago, London: University of Chicago Press (Kindle file).

Obeyesekere, Gananath. 1990. *The work of culture: Symbolic transformation in psychoanalysis and anthropology*. Chicago: University of Chicago Press.

Pearce, W. Barnett. 1994. *Interpersonal communication: Making social worlds*. New York, NY: Harper-Collins.

Pearce, W.B. 2005. The coordinated management of meaning (CMM). In *Theorizing about intercultural communication*, ed. William Gudykunst, 35–54. Thousand Oaks, CA: Sage.

Pearce, W.B. 2007. *Making social worlds: A communication perspective*. Oxford, UK: Blackwell.

Pestalozzi, Julia. 2003. The symbolic and concrete: Psychotic adolescents in psychoanalytic psychotherapy. *The International Journal of Psychoanalysis* 84(3): 733–753. doi:10.1516/G6AC-WEHN-EBWM-5VD9.

Pierre, Bourdieu. 1992. *The logic of practice* (trans: Richard Nice). Stanford, California: Stanford University Press.

Sabat, Steven R. 2006. Mind, meaning, and personhood in dementia: The effects of positioning. In *Dementia: Mind, meaning, and the person*, eds. Julian C. Hughes, Stephen J. Louw, and Steven R. Sabat. Oxford: Oxford University Press.

Scambary, James, Hippolito Da, Gama, and Joao, Barreto. 2006. A survey of gangs and youth groups in Dili, Timor-Leste. AusAID. http://researchbank.swinburne.edu.au/vital/access/manager/Repository/swin:15937.

Seligman, Rebecca. 2005. Distress, dissociation, and embodied experience: Reconsidering the pathways to mediumship and mental health. *Ethos* 33(1): 71–99.

Seligman, Rebecca, and Laurence J. Kirmayer. 2008. Dissociative experience and cultural neuroscience: Narrative, metaphor and mechanism. *Culture, Medicine and Psychiatry* 32(1): 31–64.

Silove, Derrick, and Zachary Steel. 2006. Understanding Community psychosocial needs after disasters: Implications for mental health services. *Journal of Postgraduate Medicine* 52(2): 121.

Silverman, Julian. 1967. Shamans and Acute Schizophrenia. *American Anthropologist* 69(1): 21–31. doi:10.1525/aa.1967.69.1.02a00030.

Sontag, Susan. 1988. *Illness as metaphor and AIDS and its metaphors*. NY: Farrar, Straus & Giroux.

Taylor-Leech, Kerry. 2008. Language and identity in East Timor: The discourses of nation building. *Language Problems and Language Planning* 32(2): 153–180. doi:10.1075/lplp.32.1.04tay.

Thompson, Jennifer Jo, Cheryl Ritenbaugh, and Mark Nichter. 2009. Reconsidering the placebo response from a broad anthropological perspective. *Culture, Medicine and Psychiatry* 33(1): 112–152. doi:10.1007/s11013-008-9122-2.

Toome, Emily. 2012. "Filling Wounds with Salt": The pathologisation of trauma in Timor-Leste. In *Local-Global, traversing customary community and modern nation-formation in Timor-Leste,* ed. Damian Grenfell, vol. 11, 24–30.

Traube, Elizabeth G. 1986. *Cosmology and social life: Ritual exchange among the Mambai of East Timor*. Chicago: University of Chicago Press.

Traube, E.G. 2007. Unpaid wages: Local narratives and the imagination of the nation. *The Asia Pacific Journal of Anthropology* 8(1): 9–25. doi:10.1080/14442210601161724

Ugarte, Eduardo. 1992. Running amok: The "demoniacal impulse". *Asian Studies Review* 16(1): 182–189.

Watzlawick, Paul, Janet Beavin Bavelas, and Don D. Jackson. 2011. *Pragmatics of human communication: A study of interactional patterns*. USA: W. W. Norton & Company Pathologies and Paradoxes.

West, Marcus. 2007. *Feeling, being, and the sense of self: A new perspective on identity, affect, and narcissistic disorders*. UK: Karnac Books.

Wilce, James M. Jr. 2004. To "speak Beautifully" in Bangladesh: Subjectivity as Pāgalāmi'. In *Schizophrenia, culture, and subjectivity: The edge of experience*, eds. Janis Hunter Jenkins and Robert J. Barrett, 196–218. Cambridge, UK: Cambridge University Press.

Wilson, David Sloan, and Edward O. Wilson. 2008. Evolution "for the Good of the Group": The process known as group selection was once accepted unthinkingly, then was widely discredited; It's time for a more discriminating assessment. *American Scientist*, 380–389.

Worsley, Peter. 1987. *Trumpet shall sound: A study of 'Cargo' cults in Melanesia*, 2nd ed. New York: Schocken.

Xiao, Zeping, Heqin Yan, Zhen Wang, M.D. Xu, Zheng Zou, M.D. Chen, M.D. Zhang, Colin A. Ross, and Benjamin B. Keyes. 2006. Trauma and dissociation in China. *American Journal of Psychiatry* 163(8): 1388–1391. doi:10.1176/appi.ajp.163.8.1388.

Chapter 5
An Integrated Model?

5.1 Are Constructs of Dissociation and Psychosis so Different?

An underlying proposition of the argument developed so far is, at least as far as brief psychotic presentations are concerned, that psychotic symptoms remain understandable through psychological (traumatic–structural and psychoanalytic) models of dissociation. Indeed implicit in our argument is that constructs of dissociation and psychosis are overlapping—both, after all, presuppose a mental model of failed integration. Here we review the basis for this proposition more thoroughly before going on to think about links between brief and chronic psychosis, and the mediation of culture.

In questioning the received distinction between psychosis and dissociation, critically minded nosologists have marshalled their arguments and evidence from several quarters, to include.

5.1.1 Overlapping Constructs

Experimental studies, which have shown that psychological measures of dissociation and psychosis cannot be readily distinguished—that is they do not have convincing *differential* construct validity (Moskowitz et al. 2005). To some extent this is common sense, since by definition, descriptions of both, speak of a failure of integration of different psychic mechanisms. Indeed, historical analysis of changing diagnostic trends, which demonstrates a waning in the popularity of Multiple

J. Rodger and Z. Steel, *Between Trauma and the Sacred*,
Cultural Studies of Science and Medicine, DOI 10.1007/978-3-319-24424-2_5

Personality Disorder (MPD—now termed Dissociative Identity Disorder (DID)) at the time that the diagnosis of schizophrenia began to gain ascendance, has been argued by some commentators to have been no coincidence (Gainer 1994; cf. Rosenbaum 1980). Further supporting this conflation is the recognition that patients with a diagnosis of DID have, as a group average, significantly more First Rank Symptoms (FRS) than patients with a diagnosis of schizophrenia (Ross et al. 1990) for whom FRS were historically a key and exclusive signifier, given due weight in ICD-10 and DSM-IV's criteria for schizophrenia (Nordgaard et al. 2008), and only recently downgraded in DSM-5. Ross (2008, 2014) further demonstrates that contemporary operationalized criteria in DSM-IV/5 and ICD-10 fail to adequately distinguish DID from schizophrenia. Moskowitz (2008) has traced how Janet's model of association–dissociation not only considerably influenced the model of traumatic structural dissociation previously described, but was also fundamental to Jung and Bleuler's emergent concept of schizophrenia[1] (see Sects. 3.1.2 and 4.1.1). This included Bleuler's pathognomonic "loosening of associations" in schizophrenia, a concept appearing closely linked with Janet's "reduction in psychological tension" or loss of synthetic mental function[2] (Moskowitz 2008, Sect. 3.4).

This overlap in clinical constructs is also reflected in clinical language, for example in the description of "walled-off" or "split-off" experience in dissociation (Atchison and McFarlane 1994; Van der Kolk et al. 1996), and "sealed over" experience in psychosis (McGlashan et al. 1975). The term "split-off" is also frequently invoked in psychodynamic descriptions of psychosis (Jackson 2001) and although used in a somewhat different way to that underpinning structural concepts of dissociation, as we have seen, Freud's early writings were in fact more aligned to Janet's theories (see Sect. 3.1.4, incl. Footnote 12; Van der Kolk et al. 1996).

---

[1]If the historical link between Jung and Bleuler's original concept of schizophrenia, and contemporary understanding has been severed, this can be at least largely attributed to the move away from dynamic understandings to supposed atheoretical operational criteria, paradoxically shown to have spawned a more de-contextualized, biological understanding of disorder (Sect. 1.5.1). Such links have been preserved for dissociative disorders, which along with PTSD, are the only group of disorders where an aetiological link with trauma is assumed.

[2]For Janet extreme trauma similarly compromised the synthetic function of the mind and was taken up by Jung and Bleuler, via their model of "psychological complexes", in their theorising about the origins of psychosis and schizophrenia (Moskowitz 2008; see Sect. 3.1.2). For Jung, trauma alone could be sufficient to impair the mind's synthetic function, whereas for Janet and Bleuler, some existing predisposition, compromising synthetic ability, was supposed (Moskowitz 2008). Such tensions resurfaced in later psychoanalytic models of psychosis, between those who argued for a constitutional deficit and those for whom a psychological model of current symptomatology was sufficient (London 1973).

Furthermore even in acute psychotic states, patients often manage to maintain a reality-orientated aspect of their personality (Sass 1995), similar to that described in dissociative conditions (van der Hart et al. 2004), enabling basic functional survival.

5.1.2 *Overlapping Treatment Goals*

While traditionally, intrapsychic integration of fragmented self-parts was seen as the goal of psychological treatment of dissociative conditions, a recent review of research outcomes for DID has suggested complete integration is only achieved in a small proportion of patients in treatment (ranging from 16.7 to 33 % across different studies; Brand et al. 2009). While full integration is clearly linked to greater improvement, the review by Brand et al. (2009) indicates that significant, albeit smaller reductions in symptomatology, diagnostic co-morbidity, subjective distress, medication usage and social and/or occupational functioning (depending on the study measures) can be achieved by two-thirds of patients in treatment in the absence of full integration. However the authors also conclude that "existing evidence suggests that DID treatment needs to persist well beyond 2 years to allow for integration; thus, the follow-up intervals in the current review are generally too brief" (Brand et al. 2009, 652).

This latter assertion is interesting since while an explicit (or even implicit) goal of intrapsychic integration is now rarely counted amongst the goals of mainstream psychiatric treatment for psychosis, historically psychoanalytic based treatment for psychosis did indeed have such a focus in mind, and a time-scale of years was often required to work towards this. However demonstrating an association between an integrative recovery style and outcome in schizophrenia is more contested. This may be because the degree of self-fragmentation in chronic psychosis is too great (Scharfetter 2008), and in cases of "personality disintegration" described in schizophrenia, there is not enough residual personality for fragments to coalesce around. First onset or brief, inter-episodic psychotic states may fare better.

However as with dissociative-disorder treatment (Brand et al. 2012), individual therapists have sometimes documented much higher rates of integration (up to 50 %), "verifiable in psychodynamic, clinical and psychosocial terms" (Alanen 1997, 119) and there is increasing recognition within the therapeutic community that it can be difficult to engage psychotic-persons in traditional individual psychoanalytic therapy, and that technique may also need to be modified towards a more supportive empathic stance to facilitate engagement and use of interpretations.

Over the last 40 years clinical developments and research in Finland has been pivotal in developing a model of *need-adapted treatment* which aims to be more flexible to the patient's changing needs and wider family and social context, and with a focus on both intrapsychic and interpersonal integration. In particular, the treatment team combine a combination of both modified psychoanalytic and family-systemic approaches (the latter often preceding engagement in individual psychotherapy) and take a stance that the psychotic-person's behaviour and utterances are available to be understood. Different therapeutic modalities also aim to be integrated with each other. Need-adapted treatment also inspired the developmental offshoot of the predominantly community-based *Open Dialogue* systemic approach to new onset psychosis that has reported back astonishing reductions in transition rates to chronic-psychosis alongside low uptake (and low-dose where used) of antipsychotic medication, and high-rates of social and occupational-reintegration (Aaltonen et al. 2011; Seikkula et al. 2011). For our purposes it is significant to note that the Open Dialogue approach has concluded through its operational experience that "psychotic reactions greatly resemble traumatic experiences" (Seikkula et al. 2001, 252) and its interventions are clearly informed by the work of trauma-dissociation theorists such as van der Kolk.

We also note a burgeoning interest in either indirect or direct therapeutic dialogue with psychotic "hallucinatory voices" (Corstens et al. 2012; Hayward et al. 2009), a technique also used by trauma-therapists in the treatment of DID (Ross 2006). More research is needed in this area but a cross-over pilot-study by Leff's team (2013b) with persons with medication-resistant persecutory auditory-hallucinations, that used novel computer-assisted avatar simulations of the persons malevolent-voices, but in which subjects were coached to respond to their voices more assertively, recruiting them into a more respectful dialogue, similarly reported dramatic results after just 7 weeks of therapy,[3] and assumes patients "reintegrate the projected unacceptable part of their internal world into their psychic structure" through this work (Leff et al. 2013a, 7).

A final point in this discussion however must concern our definition of integration. As Geertz ([1974]1984, 126) long ago pointed out:

> The Western conception of the person as a bounded, unique, more or less integrated motivational and cognitive universe, a dynamic center of awareness, emotion, judgment, and action organized into a distinctive whole and set constrastively both against other such wholes and against its social and natural background, is, however incorrigible it may seem to us, a rather peculiar idea within the context of the world's cultures.

Integration, from the Western perspective, is therefore predicated on moving towards this ideal *bounded whole* but is in contrivance of understandings of personhood in many non-Western cultural contexts, including that in Timor-Leste, in which a multiplicity of selves—often denoted in externalising language—not demanding coherent *internal* synthesis is more tolerated. Indeed even some Western psychotherapists are now accepting the more modest aim of facilitating *dialogue*, rather than integration, of different self-parts, and this seems an apt guiding image for the management of dissociation in non-Western cultures, being already part of many cultural practices as we have seen.

---

[3]In particular Leff et al. (2013a, 3) describes "significant reductions in the frequency and intensity of the voices and in the disturbance to their life. There was also a significant amelioration in the perceived malevolence and omnipotence of the voices" and corresponding to an overall effect-size of 0.8. Three of 16 patients who completed the therapy reported the cessation of voice-hearing experiences altogether.

5.1.3 Overlapping Aetiology

Even the assumption of different aetiologies underlying dissociation and psychotic illness has been challenged by recent attention to the high rates of trauma, and childhood maltreatment, found in cohorts of psychotic adult patients. In particular the few prospective studies, attempting to move beyond simple association have been provoking, with some showing a clear dose-response effect between the severity of maltreatment and later risk of psychosis (Read et al. 2008). Furthermore, these studies have usually controlled for the effects of other psychosocial adversities which, while of academic interest, may artificially dilute real-world effects, since in vivo, adversity often clusters together, and those who have been traumatised and/or maltreated are at greater risk of concurrent adversity and victimisation, as well as re-traumatisation (Read et al. 2008). Such cumulative adversity has been shown to exponentially increase the risk of risk of emergent psychiatric disorder, including, although not limited to, psychosis (Read et al. 2008).

These findings are complimented by the growing interest in the neurobiology of stress generally, and childhood stress and maltreatment specifically. Research suggests that such stress and maltreatment can engender dysregulation in the hypothalamic-pituitary-adrenal (HPA) axis (Teicher et al. 2003) which in turn regulates the dopamine pathways thought to be so important in the pathophysiology of psychosis (Read et al. 2014) Some researchers have also gone on to draw parallels between the structural brain changes seen in schizophrenia and similar changes seen in the brains of maltreated children (Read et al. 2014).

Approaching this from the lower level perspective of genetics, contrary to received wisdom, even individuals with high genetic loading for schizophrenia appear unlikely to develop the disorder when adopted early and raised in favourable, stable and nurturing environments (Tienari et al. 1994). While this had led some critics to question core epistemological assumptions behind much psychiatric genetics (Joseph 2006), certainly there is increasing evidence that specific genes are harmful to the individual when raised and exposed to adverse environmental and/or interpersonal contexts, but that the very same genes may be advantageous in more favourable and supportive contexts (Belsky et al. 2009 on "plasticity genes").

Other researchers have additionally challenged the dopamine-hypothesis of schizophrenia as overly simplistic, and pointed to the diverse range of receptors and pathways, beyond dopamine, affected by antipsychotic drugs (Moncrieff 2013). Moncrieff (2013, 124), drawing on re-analysis of both quantitative and qualitative research, argues for a less-specific effect of antipsychotic medication, to a more general notion of emotional "dampening down". This does not preclude the possibility of efficacy of drugs (beyond the symbolic) on dissociative–psychotic phenomena. For example medication might still have some, at least short-term, utility in those presenting with high levels of distress with a dissociative aetiology, by increasing the level of emotional arousal required to create or maintain intrusive breakthroughs into the observing self and thereby in reducing overall distress.[4]

The psychological mechanisms by which trauma may lead to psychotic symptoms has already been discussed in our earlier accounts of traumatic–structural and psychoanalytic models, although modified by us to include an account of how cultural factors may significantly shape, and even organise, dissociative experience. If at least a subgroup of what we have come to call psychosis might be conceptualised as having a traumatic–dissociative origin, then we might be better placed to understand how the impact of social and cultural factors could differentially shape its course in different settings, including shedding light on the challenging epidemiological findings from the WHO International Studies of Schizophrenia, which while not methodologically unproblematic, have reported better outcomes for schizophrenia in developing countries (Hopper et al. 2007a). These findings remain a conundrum for psychiatry, while forming the foundation for much critical analysis by transcultural psychiatrists and medical anthropologists, regarding Western psychiatric theory and practice. With relevance to our findings in Timor-Leste, one route to considering these findings is through an exploration of the possible relationship between brief psychotic presentations and more chronic psychotic presentations, including what gets called schizophrenia.

5.2 From Brief to Chronic Psychosis and the Mediation of Culture

In addition to our hypothesis that brief-psychotic states in Timor-Leste may represent an alternative response to trauma, adversity and loss in this setting, more generally we might speculate with Stevens (1987) that higher rates of brief psychotic disorders, and the better prognosis of schizophrenia in the developing world, are in some way linked. One proposed explanation is that brief psychotic presentations are more common in developing settings, and a proportion of these are incorrectly diagnosed as schizophrenia in the WHO studies. Therefore, the arguments goes, schizophrenia *appears* to have a more favourable prognosis in developing settings (Stevens 1987). Even if correct however such a model does not

[4]Such a perspective is not incompatible, with reports by patients and clinicians, that antipsychotic medication treatment may, in some instances, result in greater emotional and interpersonal connection, rather than emotional dampening. From an attachment perspective, overwhelming emotion and need for connection, will progress through "protest" to "despair", and eventually to emotional "detachment" (Shaver and Fraley 2008, 49–50). Antipsychotic medication may reduce the level of emotional arousal to a more tolerable level, such that detachment is no longer necessary, and paradoxically resulting in a greater degree of emotional and interpersonal connection.

explain why brief psychotic presentations are more common in the first place, and over-diagnosis implies a reciprocal reduction in the prevalence of schizophrenia in the same settings, if we are to assume the a proportion of the former has been incorrectly diagnosed as the latter. This is in fact consistent with our findings in Timor-Leste of lower rates of schizophrenia and other chronic psychosis, consistent with other studies in similar settings (Saha et al. 2005). A plausible model is to see the relationship between brief and chronic psychosis as a continuum, rather than as discrete disorders, and as such the greater prevalence of brief-psychotic presentations vis-à-vis chronic psychosis in Timor-Leste might be understood on account of less diagnostic slippage from the first to the second.

Indeed within conventional neurobiological research, the acknowledgement of an overlapping genetic base for both psychosis and affective disorders, has spurred an interest in dimensional, overlapping views of this group of disorders, confirming Kraepelin's later acknowledgment that psychosis and affective disorders are often not as separate as his system of binary classification initially appeared to suggest (Regier et al. 2009). This has long been acknowledged through the concept of schizoaffective disorder, but large scale epidemiological evidence in an urban Western setting has also led to the conceptualisation of acute and transient psychotic states as a nosological bridge between the psychotic and affective spectrum, on the basis of overlapping family histories for both affective and psychotic dimensions and of overlapping symptomatology—with both psychotic and affective symptoms usually co-occurring in brief-psychotic states (Marneros and Pillmann 2004), as we have seen in Timor-Leste.

Supporting a possible sociocultural explanation of the relationship between brief and chronic psychosis (see also Sect. 5.2.3) it has been consistently found that that ATPD is a significantly more stable diagnostic entity in developing country settings verses the industrialised West (Castagnini and Berrios 2011; see Sect. 1.5). Furthermore, we have the intriguing finding that at the level of intervention, one of the outcomes from the meaning and context-focused Open Dialogue network-systemic approach to new onset psychosis in Finland has been a *reported increase in the rates of brief psychotic episodes alongside a contingent and stable reduction in conversion rates to chronic psychotic disorders* (Aaltonen et al. 2011; Seikkula et al. 2011). We would assert that this model of the relationship between brief and chronic psychosis would hold even if we had underestimated the prevalence of psychosis in Timor-Leste (see Sect. 1.6 incl. Footnote 17 for commentary on the difficulty of low prevalence disorder estimates). Indeed if early, recurrent and severe trauma is a significant risk-factor for psychosis as discussed (Sect. 2.2.1) we would expect rates of *broadly defined* psychosis to be relatively high as was the case (Silove et al. 2008). However the clear findings of increased BRR relative to chronic psychosis in Timor-Leste, and the functional advantage this seemed to carry, appears powerful testimony to the sociocultural and ecological characteristics maintaining this ratio.

While the evolution of acute and transient psychotic states to more chronic psychotic or affective disorders might be conventionally understood to reflect the playing out of an underlying genetic script, as discussed in the previous section research into gene-environment interactions suggests a more complex relationship, and a key mediatory role for the environment (cultural, material and interpersonal). Some theorists have suggested a developmental model in which brief psychotic *states* might become chronic psychotic *traits,* through repeated activation and reinforcement of associated synaptic pathways (Guinness 1992a; cf. Perry et al. 1995). Another, not mutually exclusive possibility is that acute dissociative-psychotic states may become chronic traits—or at least appear to do so, on account of recurrent activation, with increasing ease, to a growing range of associated triggers—that cannot be readily distinguished from what we conventionally understand to be chronic psychotic illness. At the very least, these processes may represent possible pathways towards the development of chronic psychotic illness.[5] To put it another way chronic psychosis may develop through repeated synaptic reinforcement and/or may be understood through the trauma model, to include the effects of the increasing generalisation of trauma-triggers, re-traumatisation (including by illness and/or treatment experience itself), other chronic stressors, social exclusion and/or responses that negate meaning, alongside anything that lowers the dissociative threshold (see Sect. 5.3, incl. Fig. 5.1).

Such a model is consistent with risk of chronicity and impairment related to duration of untreated psychosis (DUP), although there is suggestive evidence that protective factors in some cultures may outweigh the effects of prolonged DUP (Myers 2011), and that effective treatment need not always equal medication, either in combination or alone (Halliburton 2009; Morrison et al. 2014; Seikkula et al. 2011). Indeed a delay in intensive psychosocial intervention (however that is culturally construed) may lead to poorer outcomes in some important domains than that attributable to a delay in antipsychotic treatment (de Haan et al. 2003). This includes in relation to so called *negative symptoms* which, as we have seen, may reflect chronic sealing-over of affective experience, that are no doubt critical for interpersonal relating and a wider sense of motivation and agency.

In considering the evidence for the asserted better prognosis of schizophrenia in low-income countries (e.g. Hopper 2008; Myers 2011) and applying this to an analysis of possible reasons for the apparent low rate of transition from BRR psychosis, to chronic psychotic states in Timor-Leste, we accept that theorising about the putative positive impact of "culture" in such contexts has tended to lack ethnographic depth and empirical grounding, with a tendency towards stereotyping, assumed homogenisation of beliefs and practices (both between so called traditional societies and of the individuals within them) and Romanticism (Hopper 2004; Lucas and Barrett 1995). How culture differentially relates to gender, sexuality, religion, profession and other fundamental aspects of social division is rarely considered (cf. Falicov 1995).

[5]Even if we acknowledge the likelihood of more primary biologically driven psychotic states in some instances, psychologically driven dissociative processes may potentially interact with such states, through dissociation along pre-existing biological fault-lines (Kirmayer 1996).

Here the limitations of our own cultural-epidemiological study are also apparent —lacking ethnographic depth and drawing on subjects from multiple ethnolinguistic groups—in order to address these issues with greater clarity. Nonetheless, the shared characteristics of Austronesian cultures have been acknowledged by many anthropologists in the region (McWilliam and Traube 2011), and we were able to evidence, supplement and build upon, existing hypothesis to some degree, regarding the better prognosis of schizophrenia in the developing world (and our ideas about brief to chronic transition), with our observations, discussions, and interviews in Timor-Leste, to include the following key areas.

5.2.1 Attribution, Stigma, and Interpersonal Relationships

Attribution of psychotic experience to external factors might be classified as "lacking insight" from a Western *neurocentric* perspective (Hopper 1991) but paradoxically has long been hypothesized to aid recovery by medical anthropologists (e.g. Waxler 1974), by reducing personal and social culpability (Kirmayer and Corin 1998) and associated cycles of personal shame or guilt, alongside family and community incrimination (e.g. McGruder 2004).[6] While the relationship is not invariable (cf. Littlewood et al. 2007), externalised attributions have been argued to reduce stigma[7] (Hopper 1991; Myers 2011). This is important because mental illness stigma has been shown to impact negatively on multiple domains of recovery—at least in Western contexts (Yanos et al. 2008).

Externalised attributions are also argued to leave a core morally-intact self behind to continue relations with others (Myers 2011), a hypothesis which the vast ethnography of sprit possession, while not coterminous with psychosis, offers further support to (Boddy 1994). Cultures leaning towards a more sociocentric version of selfhood, "emphasizing group membership as the core of identity," may also be more tolerant of idiosyncrasies in individual behaviour (providing not too

[6]Myers (2010) has further argued that North American concepts of recovery, by placing excess emphasis on personal autonomy, may increase contingent personal stress, and actually be counter-productive.

[7]Concepts of stigma have become more nuanced and sophisticated, moving away from simplistic notions of individual internalisation (although this is important), to an understanding of stigma as an intersubjective process, and operating at micro and macro-structural levels (Yang et al. 2007). However as Hopper et al. (2007b) have shown in their eloquent analysis of the impact of mental-illness stigma on marriageability in India, stigma can also be subverted and resisted, through the stubborn refusal of the family to accept "social defeat" for their afflicted kinsmen; although in China, Yang et al. (2007) provide counter-examples of family members reinforcing the stigma of their kinsmen in an effort at persevering their own moral status. Both groups of authors highlight the moral dimension of stigma. As Yang et al. (2007, 1531) put it, "by threatening what is at stake in the social world, stigma engenders what is most valued in one's innermost being"—as such the moral impact of stigma overlaps with the notion of moral injury outlined earlier in relation to trauma (see Sect. 2.3.1).

extreme or threatening) such that "individuals who are able to conform minimally may still preserve their sense of identity, belonging, and importance" (Kirmayer and Corin 1998, 204–205). Similar sociocultural characteristics are argued to contribute to enduring family support and even preservation of marriage, which in turn are argued to increase probabilities of recovery—through maintenance of moral worth, negation of the malignant effects of social exclusion and through the provision of family dialogical opportunities for understanding (Hopper et al. 2007b; Myers 2011; Tranulis et al. 2009).

Within Timor-Leste, the more obvious examples of external attributions of psychosis, were *lulik* and associated factors such as *rai nain* and/or the *fulan lotuk*. However externalised attributions were not limited to the extra-mundane, and could include—albeit usually alongside *lulik* related factors—instances of communal acknowledgement of overwhelming loss, clearly beyond the control of the individual (see Sect. 4.1.2—Case BP6). In both instances, an important factor here might be the normalisation of both cause and effect (Hopper 1991; Kirmayer and Corin 1998; Myers 2011); unseen *lulik* and associated factors are almost universally acknowledged, with the potential to impact on all members of society, whether for good or ill, and those adversely influenced were not clearly perceived as morally different to those untouched or benignly affected. Similarly in the case of trauma and loss, there were few if any in Timor-Leste unmoved by such experience. While not all who are affected by *lulik*, trauma or loss behave in a psychotic-manner, psychotic-behaviour in these contexts, is understood and validated as a possible outcome within a continuum of possible other responses. Choice of local idiom may further reinforce this tendency towards normalisation. Conceptual papers by Hopper (1991), Kirmayer and Corin (1998), and Myers (2011), all invoke Jenkins (1988, 301) work amongst Mexican-American families, which found that "a cultural preference for the term *nervios*" amongst other possible strategic framings of psychotic disturbance, evoked a more benign set of associations; possibly because *nervios* could also be used to describe non-psychotic, anxiety, mood or somatic based disturbance.

Myers (2011) reviews the use of similar inclusive idioms, in particular cross-culturally widespread terms for "excessive thinking," from studies in China and South India, and draws similar conclusions. In this regard it appears significant that a similar idiom for *excessive thinking* (Tetum: *hanoin barak*) was used to describe a range of distressing feelings, that may or may not meet diagnostic criteria for a non-psychotic presentation such as depression or PTSD (cf. Sakti 2013), but was sometimes also invoked to describe persons with evidently psychotic presentations. This term, or a narrative equivalent was indeed invoked in relation to three individuals from the brief-relapsing-remitting cohort and one individual from the AOC group[8] in addition to two other chronically psychotic individuals not included in our analysis (see Sect. 1.4.3, Footnote 11) presenting with particularly severe

[8]See Sect. 2.3.4—Table 2.1: Cases BP4, BP6, BP9 and CP4; full case histories are provided for BP4 (Emilio—Sect. 2.3.4) and BP6 (Julinha—Sect. 4.1.2).

and/or violent disturbance. This suggested this term was not reserved simply for milder cases. As with *nervios* and other cultural idioms for "excessive thinking" however it did seem to connote a respectful way of talking about such experiences. The inclusivity and low stigma attached to such idioms appear to go hand-in-hand. We might make a cross-cultural comparison with advocates of the *continuum*-model of mental illness in the West who similarly propose a reduction in stigma—mediated through normalisation—as a key advantage of this paradigm (Corrigan 2007), above and beyond its proposed greater construct validity.[9]

In addition to any bearing on stigma (and moral worth), both Hopper (1991, 318) and Kirmayer and Corin (1998) see such cultural framing as doing cultural work that in essence achieve a reduction in measures of *expressed emotion* (EE: manifesting as family *emotional overinvolvement*, *hostility* and *criticism* towards the afflicted person; Jenkins 1991, 392) High EE in families has been causally linked to poorer outcomes in psychotic patients (in particular relapse) in vast range of studies, including cross-culturally (Hashemi and Cochrane 1999). While there are exceptions to these findings, again including in transcultural studies (Hashemi and Cochrane 1999; Singh et al. 2013), Jenkins (1991) pathfinding work has since laid a new foundation for understanding how concepts of EE need to be locally culturally calibrated and may need adaption. The involvement of family members, in family cultural contexts where high levels of emotional involvement are the norm, will be experienced differently by sufferers compared to cultural contexts, where greater autonomy is expected (Cheng 2002). What may be experienced by researchers as high levels of criticism, may not be experienced as such by individuals where such behaviour does not violate cultural rules of interaction (Jenkins 1991; Subandi 2011). Notwithstanding this critique, within non-Western, low income contexts, including Timor-Leste, where living with extended family remains standard practice, the applicability of high EE (where appropriately calibrated and adapted) may be even greater given the high level of interdependency (Chakrabarti 2011).

However, the role of cultural assumptions and informed behaviours described, in responding to familial and community disharmony may achieve and maintain low levels of EE, linked to better outcomes, without the more contrived family psycho-education often needed to achieve this in Western contexts, although the latter may of course still have value, and the impact of acculturation may be undermining such local cultural effects (see Sect. 4.2.3). We did not formally measure expressed emotion (EE) within families, but our general impression was the families spoke with compassion about their relatives, with frustration more directed at healers, and occasionally ourselves as doctors, that a cure had not been found. Indeed we were obliged to abandon the administration of the family "burden of illness" interview schedule (see Sect. 1.2) early on in the course of our study, as

[9]Perhaps regrettably—at least at this level of analysis—the move towards dimensional rather than discrete, binary classification was largely forestalled for the publication of DSM-5, although it is acknowledged in the introduction to the manual that dimensional approaches to diagnosis "will likely supplement or supersede current categorical approaches in coming years" (APA 2013, 13).

it appeared perplexing to many respondents, and sometimes appeared to evoke offence.[10]

As touched upon above, the high rates of marriage (or de facto marriage) observed in the psychotic-cohort may also be relevant here (see Sect. 1.4.2—Table 1.1). Only two of entire cohort of 14 had never been married and there was one divorcee—rates of stable union far in excess of that seen in high income countries (Hopper et al. 2007b)—supportive of our impression of a high degree of interpersonal tolerance and low social stigma, although there are no doubt limits to this. Like elsewhere females appeared to fare slightly better than males in the marriage stakes[11] (although our sample size is too small for statistical analysis) and pointedly the two unmarried males were the two most violently disturbed in the BRR cohort, which may have had a bearing on marriageability. We do not have data to determine whether other males were already married at the time of onset of their psychotic symptoms, to differentiate between what Hopper et al. (2007b) call "prevention" and "disruption" effects although evidence of a disruption effect was present in the history of the one divorcee—Christiano from the AOC group, whose wife left him, plausibly because of years of his bizarre behaviour (see Sect. 1.4.3—Case CP1). In all these cases, high levels of tolerance notwithstanding, the relationship between psychotic symptoms and interpersonal rejection is, of course, likely to act both ways, and it might be the breakdown of this man's marriage contributed to his current chronic status.

The pattern of short bursts of disorganised behaviour, in the BRR group, interspersed with longer periods of functionality, might also support practicalities of relationship preservation, for as we shall see below in discussion of work (Sect. 5.2.2), even where stigma does exist, it may be trumped by performance (Hopper et al. 2007b). This is also likely holds for the AOC group, who in the main also appear to maintain some social and economic functionality. In both groups, as in other non-industrialised settings, extended family networks—themselves often emotional and culturally invested in survival of the martial relationship (particularly

[10]The exception to this rule were two a young woman, in relation to both of whom we had some suspicion of intra-familial abuse having occurred. In relation to one of these persons, our attention may have elicited further family discomfort, and perhaps even the need to discredit and disparage her (which of course could also be understood psychodynamically as placing felt "badness" in the victim and thereby recapitulating the dynamics of any abuse that had taken place—see discussion on "projection"—Sect. 3.1.1). We have chosen not to identify this case specifically but the it may be evident to the reader from the text (see Sect. 1.3—Ethics).

[11]Data reported by Hopper et al. (2007b) from the WHO-Collaborative International Study of Schizophrenia, reported rates of marriage in patients with schizophrenia from high-income countries of 38 % (28 % male, 48 % female). Reasons for gender disparity are likely complex and may be linked to both age of psychosis onset (conventionally understood to be earlier in males) and age of marriage (in many cultures this is younger in women)—both of which may have a bearing on whether adult social skills and key rites of passage (including marriage) have been successfully negotiated and consolidated before psychosis onset (Hopper et al. 2007b). Males may also present with more externalising behaviours in psychosis, itself likely partly linked to cultural scripts (see Sect. 5.2.5), which may increase the prospects of social exclusion.

if involving children), enshrined in intergroup alliances—may also support gaps in household and economic provision and this was certainly evident to some degree in some of the case histories. Even where limits to marriageability and marriage longevity exist, rejection by families of origin, or more generalized social exclusion was not observed or reported, even amongst kinsmen of potentially violent subjects. While the reasons for better outcomes in psychotic persons are complex, the hypothesis here is that such relational security may be important influence on outcome, although again the relationship likely extends both ways.

Attribution and Locus of Control Hopper (1991, 316) warns against the use of "simple-minded caricatures of how 'belief systems'...take shape, operate, and evolve over time" and externalised attribution should not be conflated with externalised *locus of control* (LOC[12]). Indeed an external LOC appeared, in one recent Western study, to predict a greater likelihood for the development of psychotic symptoms (Thompson et al. 2011), while a stronger *internal* LOC appears to be powerfully associated with recovery from psychotic illness (including for coming off antipsychotic medication) (Harrow and Jobe 2007). One way of understanding why the constructs are different is to consider that if one has a means of interacting with, and positively influencing, the externally attributed agent, then an internal LOC (so far as this concept can be culturally translated—see below) might be preserved. The ability to pacify and influence (although not control) the external agent is certainly seen in some possession cults (e.g. Boddy 1988) and a good example from the study cohort, was that of Ricardo (Sect. 2.3.2—Case BP2) who after giving back *lulik* stones, likely associated with a contract with a *rai nain* (Hicks 2004), significantly improved, and has not needed to see a healer since. While traditional healers by no means prove capable of helping all who they see with psychotic symptoms, five of the psychotic cohort in our study, reported some degree of improvement after seeing a healer (or in one case praying). Of course in the more common incidence of BRR psychosis, the very fact the condition is understood and predicted to be circumscribed in time, particularly by the timing of the new moon, confers some degree of culturally-shaped control (even if subjectively this is far from mind when in the midst of acute distress).

Neurobiological models of psychosis in the West, alongside concomitant use of medication, might be anticipated to increase internal LOC, alongside reductions in personal and social culpability and contingent stigma. That this has been shown not to be the case on all counts, might partly be understood to derive from the limited efficacy of antipsychotic medications (so a limited increase in internal LOC[13]), which

---

[12]As Harrow and Jobe (2007, 408) define it, "LOC refers to the extent to which an individual perceives events in his or her life as being a consequence of his or her actions. One may believe that events in peoples' lives result from their own efforts, skills, and internal dispositions (internal control) or that they stem from external forces such as luck, chance, fate, or powerful others (external control)."

[13]Indeed in Harrow and Jobe's (2007) prospective-cohort study a greater internal locus of control was associated with coming off medication; in theory directional causation could be either way but initial illness severity was controlled for.

themselves often have undesirable and stigmatizing side-effects (Arana 2000; Üçok and Gaebel 2008)—facts not lost on those subject to treatment in non-Western contexts (Read 2012). Somewhat counter-intuitively anti-stigma campaigns predicated on biological causation in high income countries, have in many instances, been shown to increase social stigma and public desire for social distance (Angermeyer et al. 2011). Such models may be too closely allied with the core self (also accepted to be reflected in brain biology, by individuals within Western cultures) to allay culpability, and create a sense of greater difference or Otherness. Psychosocial models of mental illness causation have in fact been shown to be less stigmatizing. However, while Hopper (1991, 316) cautions that "second thoughts might be given to 'educational' campaigns that seek to substitute 'scientific' models for local idioms of distress," psychosocial models additionally lend themselves to a greater consideration of social justice, which both local communities (Traube 2007) and social theorists (Toome 2012) have advocated for in Timor-Leste and elsewhere. Finally psychosocial models of stigma may more intuitively reflect the large effect size of social determinants vis-a vis genetic factors for psychosis.

Beyond these pragmatic arguments however, and returning to the experience and *ontogeny of self*, we might also argue that externalised attribution (whether relating to psychosocial understanding of adversity and trauma, or a greater degree of symbolic remove—as in, for example, idioms of spirit possession) and indeed the externalisation of experience itself (as seen in "hallucinations" or paranoid "delusions") may be more than simply pragmatic but act to helpfully separate out (at whatever degree of symbolic remove) the impact of trauma from a more core sense of self (see also Sect. 2.2.1)—at least as an *interim* step in recovery, rather than the victim internalising and identifying with others violent and non-contingent projections as belonging to him/herself (cf. Fonagy et al. 2002; Gergely and Watson 1999).[14]

---

[14]Indeed from both a psychoanalytic and social constructionist standpoint, further supported by new methodologies of infant observation (Stern 2003), one does not even need to invoke notions of trauma to acknowledge the experience of self is engendered (at the level of thoughts, feeling and bodily experience) through interpersonal interaction. We are intersubjective being, influenced by others and wider cultural forces. Jaynes (2000) argues that it was more social evolutionary pressure (complex societies demanding responsibility and accountability?) than ontological necessity that led our thoughts, emotions and even aspects of our bodily experience, to become experienced as personal and *belonging* to us. In our historical evolution, and arguably in other cultures (perhaps more so in pre-industrial societies) such experience may then at times appear to come from outside the self (Jaynes 2000). Contrary to Western notions of thinking as a "solipsistic activity" (Barrett 2004, 96), the work of the late Robert Barrett (2004) amongst the Iban of Borneo reminds us that some more rural, non-Western societies, embrace idioms of experience, that more closely embody its intersubjective nature. Amongst the Iban, Barrett could not easily identify a *commonly* used equivalent for the verb "to think," such that in common parlance the verb "to talk" was more commonly invoked in this context. Interesting, he also failed to find evidence of FRS amongst psychotically unwell persons in this group. To Barrett (2004, 96) FRS are axiomatic of "disorders of the privacy of thinking" within cultures who subscribe to this model of the mind. Cultures that pathologize external attribution and experience may therefore obfuscate the true intersubjective nature of self, and act to obscure the social determinants of illness, including psychosis (see also Sect. 3.1.1).

5.2.2 Work

While the relationship between social stigma and employability is no doubt bidirectional, the wider sociocultural and particularly economic context, may influence the overall direction of causality in one way or another. While the ability to contribute to household and subsistence work, and/or profitable employment, might mitigate against wider social stigma, in industrialised nations where supply of labour generally outstrips demand, the stigma surrounding mental illness may have a relatively larger impact on employability (outside of protected employment programmes), which in turn can amplify stigma (now added to by the stigma of unemployment), and the associated deleterious effects of social exclusion and malignant social positioning.

In non-industrialised nations, particularly those characterised by high levels of subsistence agriculture and the need for all family members to contribute to the upkeep of such work, apparently low levels of stigma, such as were apparent in Timor-Leste, might partly be explained on the basis of valued contribution to the household economy. This may also act to mitigate high levels of hostile and critical expressed emotion, and contribute to the maintenance of marriage. However it is also possible that in some contexts dimensions of stigma and occupational contribution have less reciprocal influence. For example a study in India suggested that while in urban-industrial settings stigma and attitudes towards employing someone with a mental illness were tightly coupled; this was not so in rural settings, where although high and punitive stigmatising attitudes existed towards mentally ill persons, if the individual was able to work, they were not excluded from employment (Jadhav et al. 2007). The authors go on to hypothesize that the better outcomes for schizophrenia in India, and other developing countries, can therefore not be explained on account of low stigma alone and argue that the effects of stigma may in fact be less important than making a valued contribution to the household economy and community life (but see critique below, incl. Footnote 15). So how might work and recovery from psychosis be related, and what evidence is there for this?

In his *Recovery from Schizophrenia—Psychiatry and Political Economy*, Warner (2003) reviews the evidence linking employment to recovery from psychosis. Like most longer term studies in psychiatry, differentiating cause and effect, from general association is precluded by largely naturalistic study designs, although the evidence of a positive impact derived from employment activities is growing. While limited to Western contexts, Warner notes that at a macro-level, people with schizophrenia appear to do worse in economic slumps, and considerably better in periods of labour shortage. Indeed he demonstrates that before the advent of antipsychotic drugs and disability benefits, psychiatric hospital bed occupancy was largely an inverse function of employment levels (accounting for 50 % of the variance)—at least in hospitals committed to therapeutic programmes and rehabilitation—although this correlation disappeared with the widespread introduction of antipsychotic medications and disability benefits. Moving to the micro-level of local studies, researchers have consistently found that patients with jobs to go to, stay out of hospital longer, including in matched samples or when illness severity (including the severity of any ongoing symptoms) is accounted for (Warner 2003). Interestingly, even though workers may stay out of hospital for longer, comparison of ongoing symptom levels between working and non-working patients suggests the two groups are symptomatically comparable (Warner 2003), although in one of the very few randomised studies comparing paid with non-paid unemployment, paid workers showed a significant reduction in psychotic-symptomatology (Bell et al. 1996).

The significance of these findings, might be underlined by the observation that in modern Western countries the rate of employment for individuals with psychotic illness has rarely been found to exceed 15 %, whereas in our study in Timor-Leste, in both the BRR group and AOC group, the majority of persons contributed to the household economy, albeit largely at the level of subsistence agriculture and/or market selling (see Sect. 1.4.2—Table 1.1)—at least between episodes and exacerbations. While Hopper (1991) notes that more needs to be known about the patterns, types and impact of work on psychotic-persons in non-Western contexts, subsistence farming and market selling, affords the kind of flexibility and accommodation, hypothesized to maximise the economic contribution of such persons, alongside the inter-episodic nature of their disturbance. The differential impact on symptoms of paid verses unpaid (or subsistence) work shown in one North American study (Bell et al. 1996) may also be less relevant to a context where large differentials in socioeconomic equality are less apparent in the general population (although this may change rapidly with the exploitation of Timor-Leste's natural oil resources) in light of evidence that suggests increasing wealth disparity may be an independent risk factor for psychotic syndromes (Boydell et al. 2004; Burns and Esterhuizen 2008; Kirkbride et al. 2014).

In terms of possible mechanisms, work may reaffirm a sense of social value and inclusion, which is argued with some evidence, to generalise to increased family and social engagement outside of the workspace (Warner 2003). While Hopper (1991, 317) cautions against equating work as "a socially valued and supported activity" with the alienation, poor pay and working conditions often characterising low-skilled jobs in industrialised societies, we might argue that the collaborative and *necessary* contributions of psychotic-persons in contexts like Timor-Leste, corresponds more with a context where "therapeutic virtue may spring from subsistence necessity" (Hopper 1991, 305).[15] Nonetheless there are limits to this argument—beset by forces of globalisation and acculturation (see Sect. 4.2.3), traditional means of livelihood may be losing their aspirational quality, especially for the young, many of whom have set their desires on the perceived economic prizes flowing from a post-Independence state, but the rewards from which have not

[15]In this light Hopper (1991) wonders whether the impact of employment in Western studies might derive more from the absence of the even more toxic effects of institutionalisation. Similarly Warner (2003, 158) notes that the "high productivity requirements and performance ratings may be particularly unsuitable for person recovering from schizophrenia" and where unmanageable may further contribute to "social defeat"—a concept increasingly linked to the social aetiology of psychosis (Luhrmann 2007).

been so readily forthcoming (see Sect. 4.1.1). Nonetheless, contributing to the household economy will not be without any reward, both in terms of material income and the relational security of social inclusion.

Moving to more psychoanalytically informed levels of explanation, Hollan (2013, 737) argues, that work can be used to compensate, offset or re-direct attention from mental distress (for either the self or the social audience), although in some instances may be more fully engaged in the "service of healing". From a dissociative–psychosis perspective, Hollan's notion of work as an "evasion" (p. 735) or as a "cover-up" (p. 736) of distress fits neatly with the model of "sealing over" of psychotic symptoms that is now well established as a common and distinctive recovery style (McGlashan et al. 1975); we have already noted the similar concept of "walled off" distress in dissociation (Sect. 5.1.1). Conversely, work in the service of healing is arguably more consistent with an "integrative" recovery style (McGlashan et al. 1975).

Examples of "work in the service of healing," particularly for psychotic individuals, are likely to be more contested. Kirmayer and Corin (1998, 207) describe a generalised but not-uncommon scenario from a non-Western context in which "psychotic experiences are viewed as religious and individuals who are able to function well enough to parlay these experiences into work as a religious healer or ritual expert may continue to be symptomatic while enjoying an enhanced social role". Similar sublimation of distress in the service of healing (and becoming a healer) have indeed been made in relation to adversity and experiences of trauma-related dissociation in non-Western contexts (see Sect. 4.1.1; Seligman 2005). In this context in the current study, we interviewed one individual from the BRR cohort, who did indeed claim himself as a healer (although he did not charge for his services) and was recognized as such by at least some members of his community (Sect. 2.3.4—Table 2.1—Case BP8). Yet contrary to Romantic dismissals of the mental illness concept[16] he was also simultaneously recognized as *bulak* and to be affected by the *fulan lotuk* by his neighbours.

[16]Somewhat Romantic models have drawn on labelling theory and imply a position that persons diagnosed with schizophrenia in industrialised countries are misunderstood "visionaries" and would likely be recognised as shamans or prophets if living in a different time or culture (Allen 1997; cf. Scheff 1970). The converse, individually and culturally-pathologising position, is that many shamans might be diagnosable with schizophrenia (Walsh 1993) or even that so called "traditional societies are actually schizophrenogenic" (Allen 1997, 357). As Lucas and Barrett (1995, 289) eloquently point out, both extremes constitute dimensions of "psychiatric primitivism" (the first "Arcadian" the second "Barbaric")—comparable with psychoanalytic concepts of "idealisation" and "denigration"—that foreclose on balanced thought. The argument presented here and elsewhere is more nuanced. With Obeyesekere (1984, pt. 3) we recognise that the narrative "myth models" along with other sociocultural "organising" influences may sometimes fail to overcome forces of disintegration, and the pattern of BRR pattern described is itself a significantly compromised position. Yet in relation to particular individuals in some sets of circumstances we would argue that such factors may delimit "illness" progression and forestall the journey on towards chronic psychotic states, characterised by persons diagnosable with schizophrenia (see also Sect. 4.1.1).

From a psychoanalytic perspective, psychotic persons acting as healers, might be perceived to be *projecting* disowned aspects of their own personality onto others (see Sect. 3.1.1) and thereby functioning more akin to Hollan's (2013) strategies of evasion and disguise. However Harold Searles (1958), a psychiatrist with extensive experience in the psychoanalytic treatment of psychosis has noted that psychotic persons can be exquisitely sensitive to the therapist's countertransference[17]; as such it is plausible that affected persons may be able to channel this sensitivity into work as healers—becoming astute at articulating the feelings and predicaments of those that come to them for help. A third possibility of course exists, in that their own experience of understanding and managing states of fragmentation and distress, may allow them, at times of greater integration, to recognise and articulate it in others. In all likelihood strategies of evasion, disguise and in the service of healing, co-exist in such persons.

While Hollan's (2013, 733) study of work acknowledges a particular concern with "middle-class American culture" as being central to North American constructs of value and self-identity, the importance of contributing the household economy in Timor-Leste and other low-income countries has already been noted. Beyond this, we might conjecture the symbolic importance of involvement in agriculture husbandry. Indeed in the West, recent innovations in therapeutic community practice, are leading to a reaffirmation of the relationship between *nature* and therapy, with many of the "root" metaphors of psychotherapy (*grounding, nurture, growth, shedding, transformation*) lifted straight from the natural world (Haigh 2012). External engagement with the natural world might therefore simultaneously be understood as an internal nurturing engagement with the self at a safe-distance. Indeed this may be all the more powerful in cultures like Timor-Leste where the land and animals themselves are imbued with symbolic *lulik* or ritual significance, and the importance of creation valued above all (Bovensiepen 2009; Hicks 1984, 2004).

At a broader level, the individual and social narratives coalescing and enacted around the value of work might be argued to help weave together fragmented experience and enable greater toleration of associated painful affect. Finally, invoking a work-metaphor, a recent re-formulation of dissociation (Nijenhuis and van der Hart 2011, 420) has likened different dissociated parts of the self to employees in an organisation that "lacks a central management but is organized by

[17]Searles (1958) argues that psychotic persons capacity for mass projection, also leaves them vulnerable to its opposite, mass *introjection* (a concept he sees as synonymous with "incorporation" and "unconscious identification"—p. 249) on account of the gap left by their projective-evacuations. He further links this to psychotic experiences of external influence (manifesting as hallucinations, passivity phenomena, or delusions of influence) but since the process is unconscious, neither the affected person or others around him/her are aware that what the psychotic person is actually responding to is the unconscious beliefs, feelings and intentions of others. Counter-intuitively then a psychotic-person who articulates the content of his/her "hallucinatory voices," thought-insertions, or "made feelings" in a context in which it is taken as meaningful by others, may be able to function in a genuine healing capacity. Searles (1958) talks of psychotic patients helping their therapists in this very manner.

the interactions among all departments" and which can involve working together on shared goals. In this light work may provide such as shared project, able to foster dialogue and cooperation between self-parts, and may explain Hopper's (1991, 305) previously cited observation that "therapeutic virtue may spring from subsistence necessity."

5.2.3 *Dialogue with the Symbolic, Religion and Concepts of Self*

Littlewood and Dein (2013, 400), remind us of Raymond Firth's hypothesis that "non-industrial societies may be more tolerant of the symbolisations of mental illness and are more likely to engage into a successful dialogue with them." We hope we have already provided ample evidence of this process in Timor-Leste, at multiple levels. To summarise, it was our experience that family and community members were able to think about the causal factors and meaning of psychotic symptoms in their relatives, within a cultural context that facilitated explanation and articulation in both mundane and cosmological terms. Community and family members were able to hold onto, and elaborate meaning out of psychotic symptoms and distress, even when the psychotic-person was unable to do so.

We would argue that the remarkable success of the Need-Adapted Treatment and related Open Dialogue therapeutic approach in Finland—the latter shown to dramatically curtail the transformation of first episode psychotic presentation to chronic psychotic (Aaltonen et al. 2011; Seikkula et al. 2011)—might be similarly understood on the basis of exacting attention to social context and personal–social meaning, in which traumatic origins are explicitly recognised (Seikkula et al. 2001)—thereby fostering both personal and social integration. Indeed Aaltonen (1994, 97), one of the pioneers of this approach, proposed the importance of "shared psychological images through which the whole staff could integrate patients' behavior and symptoms, both symbolic and nonsymbolic."

Not unrelated to this, the very high levels of religious faith practice reported in Timor-Leste might also be argued to be protective. While religiosity can complicate psychosis, projected religious faith and practice has emerged as an important supportive relational dimension to experience (Luhrmann 2013) as well as offering a cultural frame of understanding and positioning (Corin et al. 2004), symbolically matched to the existential movements between creation and destruction that often constitute psychotic experience (Obeyesekere 1984; see Sect. 4.2.1). The dominant East Timorese religion was a syncretisation of Catholic Christianity and traditional belief and practice, but also had strong practical and symbolic affinity with the Independence movement, and post-Independence identities, suggesting it may provide an important role in processing trauma, although this would need further ethnographic exploration.

While we should acknowledge that in other cultural contexts, Catholic religious affiliation has been argued to be a risk factor for schizophrenia (Murphy 1968; Murphy and Vega 1982; Scheper-Hughes 2001)—an association not fully accounted for by other social factors—and controversially linked to Catholic attitudes toward sex and marriage, the basic premise of some such findings have subsequently been shown to be highly doubtful (e.g. Hopper 2008 commentary on Scheper-Hughes 2001). In any case to transpose such findings to Timor-Leste, even if valid in other contexts, would be highly problematic on account of vast differences in ecology, social structure and, in particular the mode of affiliation and interpretation of Catholic belief and practice—not least the syncretic incorporation of Catholic belief and practice, alongside more traditional aspects, which is likely to have significantly altered the emphasis of particular doctrines. For example, high levels of "traditional marriage" and childbirth, outside of religiously sanctioned unions, were commonly described without stigma, shame or guilt.

Furthermore we might consider Louis Sass's (1992) searching thesis that the alienating and disorientating cultural *hyperreflexivity* characteristic of Western modernity/postmodernity is analogous to the loss of *taken for granted self-evidence*[18] and personal hyperreflexivity seen in schizophrenia. While the bulk of Sass' work resists the temptation of asserting a causal hypothesis, the epilogue of the work permits some exploration of this, pointing to the historical and cross-cultural record, which suggests the schizophrenia paradigmatic of Western societies,[19] was different to historical forms of psychoses described before industrialisation and cross-culturally in non-industrialised settings, which were more akin to "the more socially engaged and less bizarre forms of transient psychosis that are so common in the developing world" (p366)—consistent with our experience in Timor-Leste. He further presents some evidence, citing Guinness (1992a), of an evolution on psychotic phenomenology from the latter to the former, in first and second-generation migrants from a low to high income countries.

If the interpersonal and bodily alienation of modernity/postmodernity is therefore in some way causally linked to the nature of chronic psychotic illness seen in the West, we might contrast this with ethnographic accounts of Timorese culture (Hicks 2004; Traube 1986), which as we have seen, argue for a strong ritual-performative basis for self and interpersonal relations, that may mitigate against a hyperreflexive cognitive style. Indeed building on Sass's work, Littlewood and Dein (2013) argue

---

[18]What European phenomenological psychiatrist, Wolfgang Blankenburg, terms as "loss of natural self-evidence" (Sass and Parnas 2003, 434)—expounded on by Sass and Parnas (2003, 434) as the "loss of the usual common-sense orientation to reality, of the unquestioned sense of obviousness, and of the unproblematic background quality that normally enables a person to take for granted so many aspects of the social and practical world.".

[19]While Sass (1992, 366) would certainly not claim a unitary manifestation of schizophrenia to characterise patients in modern Western industrialised nations, he argues that the common and widely recognised "symptomatic picture involving withdrawal, highly idiosyncratic and abstract patterns of thinking, and a preoccupation with hidden meanings" is rarely described in the historical or cross-cultural accounts of pre-industrial societies.

that it is particularly the intellectual framework of the Reformed Protestant Christian church that is strongly linked to hyperreflexia and Sass (2001) himself described the shift from societies in which emotional and social life were organized around myth and ritual, to the more intellectually abstract, and disembodied ways of being and relating characterising modern society, as a particular risk-factor for this cognitive style. If anything therefore, Catholic religious practice might reinforce the more embodied ritual-performative basis of self and social relating already described. This was very much our experience of observing religious rites in Timor-Leste.

Sass' work may also shed some light on an apparent paradox: why, if symbolic capacity is lacking in psychotic persons, does the behaviour of persons with brief-psychotic presentations in this context appear socially understood, whereas the utterances of chronically psychotic persons, certainly in our own cultural context, appear idiosyncratic and obscure, requiring painstaking decoding (cf. Hopper 2008—for a bibliography of key ethnographic works attempting this). Certainly our experience with *transiently* psychotic persons in Timor-Leste was less of the obscure linguistic digressions[20] and more a matter of generally disordered speech and behaviour (see Sect. 1.4.2—Table 1.3).

This partly comes back to the holding on, and elaboration of meaning, for the psychotic individual by their family and wider community as discussed (see Sect. 4.2), but we might also again think about the psychological work that symbols do for the sufferer. Pestalozzi (2003, 741) also draws out attention to the classical distinction between *representational* and *presentational* symbols—the former including highly discursive uses of language, but the latter "always perceived as a whole…always in close connection with the object, and, owing to the sensuousness of their nature, never far removed from the emotional realm." The idea of presentational symbols appears closer to classic anthropological understanding of symbols, for example, Turner's (1967) concept of symbols having an ideological-social and a sensory-emotional pole (see Sect. 3.1.2), and again may bestow symbols with greater efficacy in such settings, to engage with emotional extremes, and thereby delimit overwhelming experience, including dissociation–psychosis (cf. Obeyesekere 1984 on "myth models"; Sect. 4.2.1). The return of brief-psychotic subjects to states of normal functioning, suggests a return of symbolic functioning, and therefore the more discursive and obscure deviations from the meaning of public symbols, may never have enough time to develop. We might also understand this on account of a continuing connection between emotion and symbol in brief-psychotic states (with emotion also indexing a shared connection with others) where as in chronic deficit states, often characterised by "negative symptoms," the anchorage between emotion and symbol becomes adrift or severed completely, and symbolic utterances may become increasingly abstract and removed from any shared emotional world.

[20]While more obscure linguistic digressions were apparent to some degree in the smaller number of more chronically psychotic persons, this too requires careful cultural calibration (see Sect. 1.4.3—Case CP1).

5.2.4 Availability of Therapeutic Pluralism

In his seminar ethnography of treatment and healing of mental illness in Kerala, India, Halliburton (2009) compares the efficacy and patient experience of Ayurvedic medicine, Western psychiatry and religious healing, for patients suffering from severe forms of mental illness requiring inpatient treatment. While methodological limitations are acknowledged, he provides compelling evidence that—even for those experiencing psychosis—a treatment modality found to be effective by one patient, may be unhelpful for another. He concludes that one of the reasons for the better outcome of schizophrenia in low income countries, may be on account of the availability of therapeutic pluralism, subsuming both traditional and modern interventions. Within the framework offered here we might further propose this to reflect the sufferers' intuitive gravitation towards the forms of symbolic healing that are most resonant with their lived experience

This was certainly our experience in Timor-Leste. Families and persons may seek help from traditional healers, trauma-based interventions (through NGOs), and emerging mental health services, according to intuited needs, availability and finances. Our limited data support Halliburton's hypothesis. Combining both psychotic cohorts, only one had never consulted a traditional healer (perhaps in this instance, because the problem seemed clearly physical having started with a head injury, albeit described to be worse during the *fulan lotuk*). For many, it was unclear whether their experience with healers had been helpful (at least for any length of time) but some were clear it had not been. Accounts from four of the documented cases (all from the BRR group) left no doubt of the sufferer's/family's perspective that intervention by a healer had resulted in significant and sustained reduction in distress. Conversely, two accounts were equally clear that the afflicted had got worse following such an intervention.

Of course, within the realm of interventions provided by traditional healers, there is likely to be wide heterogeneity and we do not have data to further break this down, although one person, from the AOC psychotic group, reported being helped by praying at the Traditional Chinese Church. While access to Western medical treatment had been limited, it was steadily increasing with the work of the fledgling East Timor Mental Health Service, and seven individuals had consulted Western doctors or nurses, either through this service or elsewhere. Only two were unequivocally clear that the consultation or intervention had helped (one being the lady with the history of head injury); two were equally clear that it had not, but four anticipated that they would soon start to take Western medicine, or would like to have the opportunity to do so.

Where, in our experience persons did take antipsychotic medication, they were unlikely—whether because of lack of access or availability, or because their symptoms settled—to take it for more than a month or two. However given emerging evidence implicating *long-term* antipsychotic use with poor outcomes and chronicity in some setting (Harrow and Jobe 2007; Whitaker 2010; Wunderink et al. 2013) this may have averted potential harmful exposure.[21]

The importance of choice in treatment, within Western psychiatry, is of course being increasingly recognised—as, for example, enshrined in all of the treatment guidelines for psychiatric disorder produced by the National Institute for Health and Clinical Evidence (NICE) in the UK. However there is little consensus or data, as to duration of treatment for brief-psychotic presentations, which lie outside of the conventional evidence base (Marneros and Pillmann 2004). Whether the impact of acculturation discussed (Sect. 4.2.3), may have in fact, resulted in some loss of efficacy of interventions by traditional healers, may be a further factor to consider.

5.2.5 Cultural Scripting of Disorder and Expectations of Recovery

The notion that even psychotic illness may play out a cultural script, in terms of expected behaviour, level of disturbance, duration and expectation of recovery, has long been noted in the medical anthropological literature (Hopper 1991; Waxler 1974), and can be understood in light of the model of dissociative-psychosis documented herein, and the dialectical tension between organising and disorganising factors within those presentations. While it finds support in our findings of high rates of brief psychotic (albeit recurrent) episodes and comparatively low rates of chronic disorder, it of course difficult to disentangle whether cultural expectations reflect observed realities, or whether they produce them. As with Geertz's (1973, 93) model of culture as a "model of and for reality" it is likely that both reciprocally constitute each other. In this context, a society like Timor-Leste with high levels of BRR psychosis, become accustomed to recovery, and yet equally often expects periods of relapse, that *importantly*, are not seen as catastrophic. In contrast the nosological positioning and validity of brief psychotic episodes has often been contested in Western psychiatry, and clinically, in our experience, such presentations are often regarded with prognostic pessimism. Again whether as cause or consequence of such cultural (and professional cultural) expectations, it is significant that studies have generally found the diagnostic stability of transient psychotic disorders (e.g. of ATPD) to be greater in developing countries compared to the developed settings (see reviews: Castagnini and Berrios 2011; Singh 2011).

[21]While much of this work is inferential (although taken together quite compelling—cf. Whitaker 2010), the one randomised, prospective study, of antispsychotic treatment for first episode psychosis (Wunderink et al. 2013) provided evidence that those who discontinued antipsychotic treatment after 1 year, fared better *functionally*, than those who maintained treatment for the 5 years of the study. While symptom levels were similar between groups, in a low-income country such as Timor-Leste, functional advantage, is likely to be critical.

Further evidence supporting the idea of cultural scripting, within presentations of brief psychosis, emerge also within the historical record. In the late 19th and early 20th century brief psychotic episodes were more widely acknowledged and legitimated in psychiatric theory, and indeed the concept has a rich historical pedigree (Pillmann and Marneros 2003). Yet the parallel evolution of various European nosological discourses is associated with subtle differences in proposed manifest phenomenology, course, and associated aetiology. While this could of course simultaneously reflect a combination of local social and ecological factors with a bearing on presentation and course, alongside theory driven observer bias, if such experiences were in fact dissociative in nature, we would expect the theory and expectation surrounding such experience to itself function as a cultural template—further patterning and shaping such experience in structure, content, time and space, and suggesting ways in which it may become resolved.

An ecological framework would also predict a reciprocal and adaptive interaction between the environment and the cultural belief system (or local ethnopsychiatric theory) that grow up around it. It is therefore of interest that attempts to unify these wide ranging historical and cross-national observations on this subject into contemporary universalistic meta-category, such as ICD-10s *acute and transient psychoses*, appear to be associated with a weakening in descriptive and predictive validity, vis-à-vis some of the earlier concepts from which they were derived (Pillmann et al. 2000; Pillmann et al. 2003).[22]

In this context the role of gender (rather than biologically defined sex) is also of interest here. In Western settings the gender distribution of presentations of brief psychotic states is skewed heavily towards females (Marneros and Pillmann 2004; Susser and Wanderling 1994), whereas in many non-Western contexts, a more equal gender distribution, comparably with Timor-Leste, has been found (Motjabai et al. 2000). Additionally while as discussed there appears to be notable variation in diagnostic stability of transient psychotic disorders between Western and non-Western settings, differential diagnostic stability of brief psychosis according

[22]For example, the enduring concepts of *bouffée delirante*, *cycloid psychoses*, *reactive/psychogenic psychoses* and *atypical/Mitsuda psychoses*—as historically developed in France, Germany, Scandinivia and Japan respectively, but now contemporaneously operational both within and outside of the geographical boundaries in which they were first formulated and influential (Pillmann and Marneros 2003)—is unlikely to be just testimony to national pride and resistance to the globalising implications of international classification, but may reflect a closer "goodness of fit" with the culturally and ecologically shaped needs of the local population. The predictive value of DSM-IVs Brief Psychotic Disorder has been subject to less empirical comparison with such local concepts, but when compared to ICD-10's Acute and Transient Psychosis, has been found to be too narrowly defined in terms of duration and failing to address affective dimensions of such presentations (Pillmann et al. 2002).

to gender has been rarely examined.[23] While not necessarily typical of wider findings in other respects, one study in the United Kingdom found that significantly more men with ATPD went on to develop chronic psychotic disorders than women (Singh et al. 2004). While weighted family histories may have accounted for some of this, and there is a renewed appreciation of poorer outcomes for psychosis in men, across different sociocultural settings presumed to be on account of biological difference (Aleman et al. 2003), such observations also need to be explored in light of differential (both pre- and post-morbid) social perceptions and expectations of men and women, differential access to social and psychiatric roles, and differential community perceptions of disordered behaviour and threat in the two genders, that may shed light, beyond biogenetic differences on, these findings (cf. Burns 1992; Nasser et al. 2002; Piccinelli and Homen 1997). This would require further ethnographic work in relation to our findings in Timor-Leste, although both Hicks (2004) and Traube (1986) have documented important differences in gender role that may be relevant to our discussion. In particular women are seen to be more aligned to the *interior* world of spiritual authority, with men more aligned with the *exterior* world of politics and human affairs. Traube (2011)—structures reflected in domains in which psychotic behaviour takes place (cf. Littlewood and Lipsdege 1987; see Sect. 4.2.2)

5.3 An Integrated Model

In this work we have drawn on a range of diverse literatures, from Janet and the contemporary theories of structural-dissociation he inspired (Chap. 2), through Freud and the psychoanalytic tradition (Chap. 3), and onto anthropological and narrative ideas (Chap. 4). We have attempted to bridge theories focused on the individual, with theories more aligned to sociocultural and political context, in which individuals act and are embedded. It is unclear if these theories can be commensurate or indeed if integration is desirable or possible. It may be that particular theories are more akin to paradigmatic lenses for privileging selective aspects of reality to bring into focus particular ways of understanding. While throughout the work we have attempted some integration and synthesis—summarised below in its key aspects—there remain uneasy points of disjuncture, in

[23]Direct comparison across groups is further complicated by different definitions of brief psychosis. One such construct—Non-Affective Remitting Psychosis (NARP—Susser and Wanderling 1994) has a longer duration criterion of up to 6 months and is defined a priori by an absence of relapse over 2 years (Castagnini and Berrios 2011). The terminology should not be taken to mean an absence of affective symptoms, but rather presentations that fail to meet full criteria for a major affective psychosis (bipolar or schizoaffective disorder). While different operational criteria may pick up slightly different groups with different prognostic implications, generally such constructs are overlapping, and a dissociative model would also predict a population continuum in relation to number of symptoms, severity and duration.

particular between agentic and deterministic accounts of individual experience and behaviour. According to Littlewood (1996, 34) this is both predictable and inevitable since such competing accounts "generally reduce one position to the other as prior and essential" (see Sect. 1.7.2).

We have outlined how predisposition to dissociative experience (including psychotic symptoms) may relate to predisposing personality traits, early childhood experiences of trauma (potentially manifesting in a "disorganised attachment" strategy) and a cultural context in which dissociation is socially learnt and/or tacitly sanctioned as a possible coping strategy (Sect. 3.1). Culturally adaptive dissociative states may however increase the risk of non-adaptive "pathological" states (Kirmayer 2011) and in this context we argue that later adult trauma, can precipitate or exacerbate dissociative-fragmentation in self-experience, as set out in the model of structural dissociation (Sect. 2.2). Fragmented, affect-laden, experience related to trauma may be sealed-over, but in response to specific triggers, may break through into conscious awareness—decontextualised from their traumatic-origins—and manifest as psychotic-symptoms (Sect. 2.2.1) such as hallucinations or passivity phenomena. Paranoid thoughts may represent a generalisation or specific-focus of trauma-related hypervigilance and/or apparently delusional beliefs may derive from attributions made by the afflicted person in response to the kinds of decontextualized anomalous experience described. In the sealed-over state, affect-laden aspects of self are not available to the individual, and the ensuing emotional-deficit state provides one possible model of so called negative symptoms, apparent to others.

In bringing in culture, an early guiding image we had was that traumatically fragmented pieces of self might be shaped and contained by local cultural beliefs and practices (including unconscious cultural scripts of behaviour) somewhat like *grains of sound* poured into and contained within a *mould*. We have argued that a fragmented-self may indeed be more susceptible to cultural-shaping—albeit in a rather immediate and concrete way—in essence using culture as a kind of carapace or scaffold, in the absence of more internalised coherence (Sects. 3.1.4 and 4.2.1). The fragmented self is of course not really like grains of sand, but perhaps more akin to polarised elements with one pole indexing internal drives, conflicts and emotions, and the other pointing outwards towards significant others and wider community (towards or about whom of course drives, conflicts and fantasies may be directed or concerned).

According to a convergence of both anthropological and psychoanalytic models, *cultural symbols*—with their physiological-emotional pole and their social-moral pole (Turner 1967; see Sect. 3.1.2)—would then provide the "glue", allowing these polarities to be held in tension and aligning fragmented bits of self loosely within this cultural mould. Symbols may be further woven into *narrative* (arising out of the relationship between symbols) and whether consciously held ("stories told") or simply enacted ("stories lived"; cf. Pearce 2007), culturally endorsed narratives may provide further stability for states of sealing-over, and explain why some individuals do not suffer with intrusive traumas and/or related psychotic symptoms (Chap. 4). Conversely where narrative falters or the gap between "stories lived" and "stories told" becomes too great, dissociation–psychosis may ensue (cf. Kirmayer 1996; Sects. 4.1 and 4.2.1).

Symbols and emergent narratives may therefore be seen as an important *container* of progenitorial psychotic states. However symbols may also be a *trigger* of psychotic states. We have argued that traumatic experience may become associated with cultural *symbols*, from the moment of encoding into memory, such that the same or related cultural symbols—in the case of Timor-Leste, connected to local understanding of spirit-sacredness and taboo (*lulik*) and associated areas—may be sufficient to trigger a breaking through of sealed-over, affect-laden aspects of self or traumatic-experience into conscious awareness (Sect. 2.3).

While the model of structural dissociation views psychotic phenomena such as hallucinations as "echoes" of past traumatic experience (Sect. 2.2.1), psychodynamic models also allow for them to be additionally sometimes understood as projections of intolerable aspects of self (that may nonetheless be related to trauma) onto others (or as the outcomes of other "primitive defence mechanisms"; Sect. 3.1). Furthermore psychodynamic theories of symbolism, usefully combined with anthropological models, permit the re-working of both traumatic experience and internal *phantasy* in compromise formations bridging the intrapsychic and the interpersonal (Sect. 3.1.2)—which may be creative or conservative/regressive (the latter for example where conforming to illness models; Sect. 4.2.3).

A breakdown in the capacity to symbolise however might be a precipitant that leads to psychosis—[symbolic] representation may be conflated with reality in psychotic worlds (Sect. 3.1.2)—just as traumatic-flashbacks are experienced as belonging to the present rather than the past (Sect. 2.1.2). The paradoxical significance of the *fulan lotuk* however is that, if as we propose the moon is a symbol that is "good to think" with (Ortner 1973, 1341; Sect. 3.1.2), its absence during the new/crescent moon period, may resonate with or even compound a loss of symbolic capacity and contribute to an ensuing psychotic state of mind, in persons' whose symbolic capacity is already compromised—including by trauma (Sects. 4.1.1 and 5.1.1, Footnote 2). However, whatever its more rooted influence on the capacity to think, the psychotogenic potential of the *fulan lotuk* may also have subsequently become culturally scripted (and therefore expected and predicted) over time. From an observer's perspective the "symbol" of the *fulan lotuk* might be seen, paradoxically, to *symbolise the absence of symbolism.*

However the community around the psychotic-individual appeared able to hold onto, and elaborate on, an understanding of meaning, in relation to what is being expressed—both at a mundane (e.g. related to trauma and loss) and symbolic *lulik* level (Sects. 3.1.2, 4.2.1, 4.2.2 and 5.2.3). We have argued that the ability and willingness of significant others to symbolise the sufferer's experience, provides an important means of containment and validation of the deeply felt realities of the psychotic-person, buying time for the return of the afflicted person's own symbolic-capabilities, and helping them move to a position of recovery and restoration to the community (in contrast to the malignant social-positioning of their experience and personhood, faced by those who experience psychosis in the West). Alongside this, cultural scripts of behaviour and understanding may delimit such a breakthrough in time and space, permitting distress to be communicated and understood but then sealed-over once more and facilitating the individual's return, adaptation and survival in their local community.

The effectiveness of symbolic forms in containing psychotic–dissociated states, while articulating underlying meaning and distress, will depend on the resonance of such symbols with conscious and unconscious meaning and affect-laden experience (alongside their wider social valence), and as Obeyesekere (1984, pt. 3) notes in his discussion of "myth models" will not always succeed. Our discussion of cultural revitalisation however provides a context in which the healing efficacy of cultural symbols may become rejuvenated (Sect. 4.2.3). This process can be innovative or conservative, although in the context of our study was mainly the latter.

5.3.1 Predisposing, Precipitating and Perpetuating–Recovery Factors

In Fig. 5.1, we have attempted to draw together various factors contributing to either psychic integration–recovery or disintegration–psychosis, within a fairly conventional *bio-psycho-social(cultural)* framework, incorporating predisposing, precipitating and perpetuating (or resolving) factors. Such factors might be fixed (and even innate) or acquired and dynamic (along a spectrum of malleability). Within the diagram, we have tried to indicate whether a particular factor is fragmentary and psychotogenic-(encircled in black) or integrative and adaptive (encircled in white), with shadings of grey indicating either the potential for adaptation or harm (Fig. 5.1a) and/or from lesser to greater degrees of psychic-disintegration (represented by increasing shading of grey; Fig. 5.1c). There is clearly some overlap between predisposing, precipitating and perpetuating factors, and indeed many predisposing and/or precipitating factors (including primary biological ones[24]) can be conceived as simultaneously lowering the threshold for the breaking through of sealed-off aspects of self-experience once dissociation is established. Similarly

[24]As with states of dysphoria (see Sect. 2.3.4, incl. Footnote 17) similar ideas, able to acknowledge and incorporate a role for organic factors, were established in the models of psychogenic psychosis expounded by Wimmer and other Scandinavian psychiatrists (Castagnini 2010). In our model acute organic factors, such as infection and nutritionally deficit states (clearly common in Timor-Leste) alongside potentially lifelong subtle neurodevelopmental deficits (which may itself derive from pre-natal maternal malnutrition or infection—Piccinelli and Homen 1997)—for example in language (Rubio et al. 2012), processing speed and associated memory (Leeson et al. 2010)—might lead to overload or reduce the coherence of neuropsychological systems, and their ability to maintain dissociative seals, leading to breakthrough of disorganised and emotive traumatic experiences. It is possible the pattern of neurodevelopmental deficits shown to be risk-factors for psychosis in high-income countries, differs to that seen in low-income countries, on account of different infection-profiles and differing possibilities in obstetric/neonatal care which may be significant.

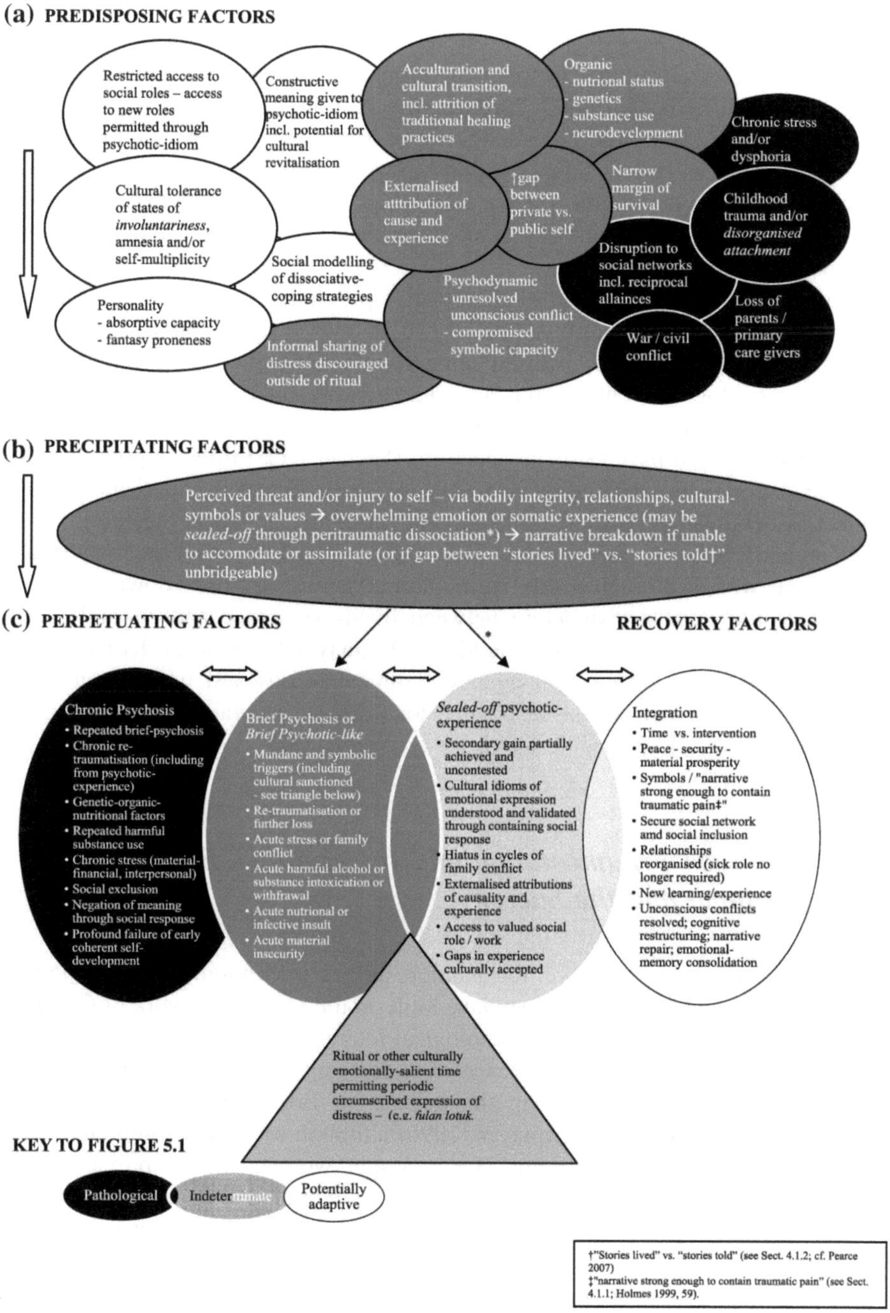

Fig. 5.1 Pathways to dissociative psychosis and recovery in Timor-Leste

potentially adaptive predisposing sociocultural factors might overlap with potentially integrating-recovery factors.

Predisposing sociocultural factors with strong potential for adaptive functioning (Fig. 5.1a—white background) include dissociation as a socially learnt and culturally-valued coping mechanism, the cultural tolerance of narrative multiplicity and social spaces that allow relationship and identity negotiation through dissociative-psychotic idioms. These could link with genetic factors, expressed through "plasticity genes" (Belsky et al. 2009; Sects. 3.2 and 5.1.3), in the context of gene-environment interactions.

Figure 5.1b details a model of dissociative-psychosis precipitation, which we have conceptualised as narrative-breakdown. However in so far as narrative is understood to be the fluid medium upon which existential contingencies from biology to ecological context converge, inextricably linked to and animated by emotion and sense of physical embodiment it should be clear that narrative encapsulates the bio-psycho-social spectrum (Sect. 4.1.1). From the point of view of lived experience narrative is also able to weave between experiences of the subject as being acted on (deterministic) and acting on the world (agentic). As we have argued narrative may be violated through attacks on values, beliefs and symbols, as well as through bodily-harm. Narrative may also breakdown simply on account of too great a disjuncture between lived-experience and cultural ideals, between "stories-lived" and "stories-told" (cf. Kirmayer 1996; Sects. 4.1 and 4.2.1). All trauma violates agency, but agency (both conscious and unconscious) also influences how trauma will be responded to. Restored or realigned narratives are acknowledged as a key specific factor for recovery.

5.3.2 Between Fragmentation and Integration—Between Trauma and the Sacred

In offering a dynamic, multilevel formulation, able to incorporate a range of factors from the biological to the social, we have built on the pioneering work of Guinness (1992a, b) who argues for psychopathological interaction between states, traits and events—including gender, the presence of underlying mood or anxiety symptoms and magnitude of life events—in the genesis of brief-psychotic presentations. However as summarised by Kirmayer (1996) although such interactions may give rise to apparently distinct groups (for example women with depressed mood responding to apparently minor life-events) we would additionally frame such factors within a larger matrix of influences tipping the balance one way or the other in the interplay between integration and disintegration (Fig. 5.1). For example, dysphoric states and general social stress (however culturally conceived) may be argued to tip the balance towards fragmentation (see Sect. 2.3.4, incl. Footnote 17), while the gender of the person experiencing psychosis may influence the expectation and response of others (with men arguably being likely to be perceived as more dangerous) and thereby influence contingent illness roles available to those manifesting high states of distress (Sect. 4.2.2 and 5.2.5). The progression from brief psychotic episodes to more chronic psychotic states is argued to depend on a range of mediating factors that either prolong the assault on emotion, body and self, or allow for respite and resolution. Where chronic disorders develop, they may still exist in a dynamic state of greater or lesser organisation–dissociation and be prone to exacerbations as described, in response to culturally symbolic triggers. Even if a distinct primarily biologically driven psychotic state was confirmed (as, for example, in the case of, Lorena, an elderly woman with dementia and psychotic-symptoms secondary to head-injury; Sects. 1.4.3 and 2.3.4—Table 2.1: Case CP4) organic states of disintegration and confusion are embedded and overlap with the psycho-cultural process described (see Sect. 5.3.1, Footnote 24; cf. Kirmayer 1996) leading to exacerbation at the time of the *fulan lotuk* or other culturally salient times or places.

According to Last (2000, 380) it is often "not 'healing' in any complete sense that is being sought" by survivors of conflict-ridden countries, "it is the means of going on living as best, as joyfully, as one can, alongside others who are not half as hurt as you are, for it is through their energy and strengths that wider recovery will occur"—"Its target is the reduction of loss to the level of an impairment that can be lived with". In this respect the recurring nature of the *fulan lotuk* appears to occupy an indeterminate space between fragmentation and organisation, illness and healing, ensuring that individual trauma and loss is revisited and acknowledged by both self and wider community, but also enabling the individual to inter-episodically function and participate, to varying degrees in the material and cultural life of his or her community.

The lunar cycle in Timor-Leste might also appear to frame, over a smaller time-scale, what the seasons of the year, for Harrison (2004, 592), eco-culturally scaffold: a to-and-fro movement "between times of closeness or attachment to these spirits (which are times also of memory and sadness), and times when the living disengage or distance themselves, so that the structure of the [lunar cycle] reflects the emotional ambivalences—of closeness and separateness, of remembrance and forgetting—that colour people's ties with the dead in these societies." This is also consistent with Truab's (1986) description of Mambai ritual cycles relating to the sacred and profane, and the living and the dead—similarly structured in relation to the seasons and less conspicuously to events in the lunar cycle (where coincident with other seasonal markers, such as the end of the dry season—see Sect. 3.1.2). Putting this psychoanalytically, Bion eschewed earlier relatively linear ideas of development and he instead described a lifelong oscillation between the potentially more consolidated and grounded "depressive position" and the more creative yet mentally dispersed "paranoid-schizoid" position (Eigen 2004; Frosh 2006). Perhaps too East-Timorese culture allows for this mental movement back and forward at culturally sanctioned times, including the *fulan lotuk*—presumably the darkness at the time of the new moon (for those who retain sufficient symbolic capacity) represents a time of reflection and consolidation (further ethnographic exploration of this would be useful).

There may however be a further paradox and inversion, in that in those persons predisposed to psychosis (lacking strong symbolic capacity, potentially on account of trauma and compromised self-development; Sects. 3.1.2, 4.1.1 and 5.1.1, incl. Footnote 2), the pain of the reflection may be too much to tolerate and rather than leading to the consolidation and integration of the "depressive position" instead triggers psychic-dispersal and psychotic-relapse.

Moreover, since idioms of dissociation also appeal to unseen cultural spiritual realities, through individual dialogue with private, public and ideal selves, "illness" might in fact be sometimes conceivably reframed as a form of cultural resistance and revitalisation (Sect. 4.2.3). To treat and label such distress through the terms of a Western illness model, particularly if reified and de-contextualised from wider influences and relationships, may unwittingly collude with early colonising agendas (Ugarte 1992). This does not mean that suffering should be ignored or that Western informed treatments may be of value. It may nevertheless need to be acknowledged that symptoms may maintain relevance until no longer required in terms of local family and community dynamics, wider cultural forces, and the search for social justice (cf. Toome 2012).

Within this model, the self can be seen to be simultaneously subject to opposing fragmentary and synthetic forces, and indeed in the patterns of BRR psychosis described, he/she appears to oscillate between states of greater and less integration over time. Within this it is unlikely that an individual occupies either polarity for long, and in so far that psychosis, also becomes available as a cultural template, or idiom of distress for communicating and social positioning, psychotic states may also sometimes be more organised than they appear—in some contexts perhaps better understood as "psychotic–like". However the *biolooping* (Sect. 1.7.2) between genuine states of fragmentation, local cultural understanding and cultural templates of madness may give rise to the different culturally patterning and form (not merely content; Luhrmann et al. 2015; McLean et al. 2014) of psychotic-symptoms in different cultural and historical contexts, demonstrating the concept of *cultural pathoplasticity* (see Sects. 1.1 and 1.5).

5.4 The Question of a "Cultural Syndrome"?

The culturally patterned presentations of distress identified in Timor-Leste raises the question of whether these might be better understood as cultural-syndromes? If so what would be their defining features? At the level of symptoms we have seen there is too broad an overlap between descriptions of BRR psychotic presentations in Timor-Leste and descriptions of BPD in DSM-IV/5 (with its emphasis on *disorganisation* of speech and behaviour) and with ATPD in ICD-10 (with its emphasis on abrupt onset and evolving symptom-polymorphism) to convey a sense of local specificity in symptomatology alone. While it would be interesting to see whether any of the broad terms for madness or psychotic behaviour were statistically more likely to be linked to particular presentations (for example, whether the Tetum term *pontu*, sometimes interpreted as "talking too much," might denote "pressure of speech" and associated mania) this would require a larger sample than currently available, and it is already clear, as has been found elsewhere, that such terms are not specific (Kirmayer 1996), and there may be multiple overlapping terms that can signify psychosis or mania.

At the level of cultural understandings of aetiology, the linking of psychotic presentations to *lulik triggers* (rather than simply idioms of description), including the associated *rai nain* and the *fulan lotuk* (which could appear as cause, trigger or idiom), appears fairly specific to psychotic-states (although in journeys towards recovery the *fulan lotuk* may *subsequently* trigger non-psychotic states of behavioural disturbance: see Sect. 2.3.2—Case BP2). Again however similar brief psychotic-states have been described in other parts of the world in response to supernatural beliefs and could not be seen as unique to Timor (Jilek and Jilek-Aall 1970). Indeed this argument could extend to lunar influence, including consideration of whether the temporal-patterning of symptoms at the time of the new moon is again specific to Timor-Leste?

The perceived influence of the moon on psychiatric presentations, including psychosis, is enshrined in the historical English legal category of "lunacy," and finds expression in Shakespeare and other late renaissance literature, but has roots at least as far back as medieval times and such cultural conceptions also extend to the present day—not least amongst mental health professionals (McCrae 2011). Of interest for comparative purposes is not only was a *lunatic* legally defined in England in the 18th century by the presence of "lucid intervals…depending on changes of the moon" but also as "one who hath had understanding, but by disease, *grief*, or other accident hath lost use of his reason" (McCrae 2011, 68; emphasis added) suggesting it was culturally also sometimes linked to issues of trauma or loss. Additionally according to McCrae (2011, 47) "in medieval magic, the moon was closely linked to witchcraft" which clearly resonates with the explanatory model of lunar influence provided to us by one of key cultural consultants (Sect. 2.3.4). Furthermore although in popular culture it is now predominantly the full moon that is bestowed with such influence, the leverage of the new moon is also culturally established, including in the work of the mid-Renaissance physician and occultist Paracelsus (McCrae 2011).

Conversely there appears surprisingly little written about the relationship between the moon and madness cross-culturally, and where such associations have been made by colonial psychiatrists, for example in India (Oda et al. 2005), it is unclear whether such associations represent yet another committal of Kleinman's *category error* by the observing Western psychiatrist or an authentic reflection of spontaneous belief and behaviour. Given the likely positioning of the moon as an important *symbol for thinking* however (Sect. 3.1.2), it would be surprising if similar associations were not found to have at least some cross-cultural expression.

Empirically associations between phases of the moon and madness in secular Western contexts remain controversial, methodologically contested, and for many now discredited, yet this does not rule out the possibility that in earlier times, before the widespread availability and use of electric-lighting (Sects. 2.3.4 and 3.1.2,

Footnote 10) and before, according to Obeyesekere (1984, pt. 3), our symbols were "decoded and secularized" (Sect. 4.2.1), a stronger empirical association may have existed. Even now we might suspect that the retention of such beliefs within both popular and professional subcultures may provide a category to "act into" (cf. Pearce 2007; see Sect. 1.7.1) and in this respect it is of interest that some very highly powered studies have demonstrated associations between psychiatric presentations, including of psychosis, associated with the *new moon* (e.g. Climent and Plutchik 1977), although there remain other studies with negative findings (McCrae 2011).

Either way, as with other so called culture-bound syndromes (Jadhav 2007) there is enough uncertainty to question the assertion that symptoms and temporal pattern of the *fulan lotuk* is truly culture-bound, although of course the unique cultural elaboration of meaning and response, arguably also understandable in the context of cultural revitalisation, may be more culturally specific. While abstracting any such symptom pattern from the local context poses both epistemological issues and clinical dangers as we have spelt out, we would also resist the designation of our findings as cultural-bound for both empirical and pragmatic reasons, including a desire to minimise the risks of reification and exotification, which as with a universalising stance, can equally obscure a more nuanced sociocultural reading. We would also argue our model is both specific and general, and potentially transferable, at a general level, to other sociocultural contexts. We have expounded in detail as to how such culturally symbolic triggers may become intertwined with the mundane and painful realities of trauma, loss and adversity, but in light of the increasingly clear significance of such environmental and interpersonal risk factors for psychosis (Sect. 2.2.1) it is likely that such links could be made (to varying degrees) elsewhere, although requiring revision in light of new contexts, cultural scripts and symbolic encoding.

Even if we had argued for local specificity (for example, combining disorganised-symptomatology, culturally understood aetiology, local response and temporal patterns taken together) going on to identify its core features would pose further difficulties still.[25]

[25]This difficulty is also shared by the majority of Western-derived psychiatric disorders described in DSM and ICD diagnostic manuals, most of which rely on polythetic criteria and consequent multiple symptom permutations. Lilienfeld and Marino (Castagnini 2010) helpfully propose that many psychiatric presentations might be linked to each other through the notion of a central prototype, itself derived from Wittgenstein's ([1953]2010) notion of *family resemblances*. However since such concepts are themselves "characterized by unclear boundaries and an absence of defining (i.e., criterial) features" (Lilienfeld and Marino 1995, 416) in many cases defining the ideal prototype may itself be elusive and rather we must return to Wittgenstein's ([1953]2010, 36[e]) original concept of family resemblances—explicitly modeled on the physical and temperamental traits of closely related human kin, such that "if you look at them, you won't see something that is common to *all*, but similarities, affinities and a whole series of them at that" [italics in original].

5.5 Implications for Research and Intervention

The emergence of BRR psychotic episodes appeared to represent a culturally-shaped response to trauma, providing a fit, perhaps not only with local beliefs and ways of life, but also with the wider ecological and economic context that both enable and constrain opportunities for expression, meaning and functioning. In contrast to this complexity the practical and financial emphasis of psychiatric research in high-income countries is largely dominated by brain-research often predicated on reductionist and de-contextualised premises of mental distress. However as Berrios (2014, 38), notes: "Given that therapeutic approaches to hallucinations based on the neurobiological model have so far had limited success it is ethically incumbent upon clinicians to search for alternative ways of understanding hallucinations"—we would obviously extend this call beyond hallucinations to psychotic-phenomena in general.

We acknowledge the full implications of our model remain to be worked out and clearly further research is needed. This includes more in-depth and focused ethnography of mental illness, including psychosis, in Timor-Leste. Building on case histories, ethnographic work might follow individual trajectories over time and in context. This would be enriched by a specific focus on more fully elucidating beliefs and associations around psychotic presentations (such as the *fulan lotuk*), attendance to how emotions are expressed within families, and exploration of early development. The latter might include a focus on how children are socialised into the use of dissociative-coping mechanisms. Further empirical work is needed to attempt to grapple with the relationship between culture and dissociative coping mechanisms although this is methodologically challenging in vivo (see Sect. 1.6—Footnote 19). Possibly experimental psychology has a role, as in studies looking at induction of delusional-like experiences through hypnosis (Cox and Barnier 2010), which might be extended to compare proneness across different narrowly defined ethnic groups. Sociological and epidemiological studies looking at the responses of remitting-relapsing psychosis to changes in employment and perceived security would also be illuminating. Regarding the relationship between trauma, dissociation and psychosis, ongoing research and debate is needed to clarify the nature of these relationships (cf. Laddis and Dell 2012 vs. Moskowitz 2012), and exceptions to them. Is the trauma-dissociative pathway a subgroup of wider psychosis (cf. Ross 2008) or is the multifactorial model (which includes biological factors) presented here a robust explanation for the spectrum of psychotic presentations, in this and other cultural settings and what are the limits of its explanatory power.

Other potential areas for research are highlighted in the text and our list is by no means exhaustive. Even with further research the problem of theoretical integration and commensurability would of course remain. Given that the epistemological sands of psychiatric theory and practice are forever shifting, the utility of a model often comes from its heuristic and clinical utility. Much psychiatric progress has been driven by noting response to intervention, although this should not lead to reification of hermeneutic models.

While Freud argued that therapeutic work with delusions would "consist in liberating the fragment of historical truth from its distortions and its attachments to the actual present day and in leading it back to the point in the past to which it belongs" this remains an *Occidentocentric* perspective on trauma, and the tension in understanding the "work of culture" in Timor-Leste and other cultural contexts is appreciating that efficacy may in part rely on sustaining a degree of "symbolic remove" from mundane realities. Recovery factors promoting "sealed off" psychotic-experience are outlined in the text and summary (Sect. 5.3, incl. Fig. 5.1c) above and include externalised attribution of cause and experience, related cultural tolerance of *gaps* in reported experience (Kirmayer 1994) and the community's ability to hold onto meaning. The "cultural efficacy" of such understanding may be at risk of erosion from further Western acculturation, potentially leading to the unsealing of psychotic-distress and the march towards chronicity. Nonetheless as our work and others attests to, symbolic and more mundane understandings of psychotic-phenomena, can co-exist and may be invoked by afflicted persons and other local stakeholders, in different times and contexts, in keeping with the pragmatic demands of the situation (cf. Young 1982). We have also noted the potential for cultural revitalisation, whether through the invocation of traditional illness idioms or otherwise.

An obvious framework for thinking about sites of intervention would be to make reference to the "recovery factors" *promoting integrated experience* also outlined in the text and summary above (Sect. 5.3, Fig. 5.1c). As with considerations of the nature of mental distress, modalities of intervention might also be divided into "naturalistic" and "personalistic" focused solutions (cf. Littlewood 1996; see Sect. 1.7.2). Examples of the former might include structural interventions focusing on security, job creation, housing and wider infrastructure development (cf. Silove 2005). In contrast personalistic-interventions attend directly to experience, relationships and meaning. Some interventions clearly straddle both aspects, and indeed structural interventions are arguably important in so far as they promote *felt security* and facilitate agents to pursue their goals, whether material, relational or existential. This could include medication, which may have a direct, independent effect on neuropsychological pathways but of course also influences meaning, at both individual and sociocultural levels. Assessment of the effect of different medications on distress, coping and personal agency is complex, and needs to include a consideration of both short and longer term effects.[26]

[26]Medication may also have a role for those in severe distress and finds some support in the wider literature (Marneros and Pillmann 2004). We only received feedback from one person in the psychotic-cohort who were seen by the local mental health service during the time of our study in whom low dose antipsychotic medication appeared to reduce levels of recurring distress. More generally mental health workers described the use of low dose medication, including in psychosis—whether symptom remission was really on account of pharmacological activity, or else the validation and "placebo" healing efficacy provided by "exotic" Western medical treatment (cf. Geest and Whyte 1989) is hard to be clear on. The longer term implications of medication, for better or worse, appear less certain; however in the context of the possible wide ranging dimensions of "illness" here conjectured, would need further careful consideration (e.g. see Sects. 1.1, Footnote 5 and 4.2.3). Even at the level of direct pharmacological action some have concerns about negative longer-term effects (Sect. 5.2.4, incl. Footnote 21).

Similarly attention to social justice, called for by both local East Timorese communities (Traube 2007) and social theorists (Toome 2012), as with trauma itself, subsumes both determinism and agency. Justice requires deterministic structures and mechanisms, and if necessary incarcerates those at risk of causing continuing harm. Ultimately it is also the effect on the meaning for victims that make it so important for healing of emotional wounds; summed up in the early 20th century English legal aphorism "Not only must Justice be done; it must also be seen to be done." The fact that justice was *not* seen to be done has been highlighted as one the key factors limiting the effectiveness of the Timor-Leste Commission for Reception, Truth and Reconciliation (known by its Portuguese acronym CAVR) since perpetrators of serious crimes sought refuge and de facto immunity from prosecution within the Indonesian state that directed and was complicit in their crimes (Le Touze et al. 2005). Truth it seems was not enough, and indeed for some may have compounded the sense of injustice, anger and humiliation. Le Touze et al. (2005) go on to propose that because of the uncertain impact and strategic choices made by truth and reconciliation commissions interested and affected parties should be consulted and given opportunity to take ownership and shape the process. Along similar lines DelVecchio Good (2013) notes rituals imposed from above, may lack the efficacy of those transforming or resurrecting existing traditional models from below—although time, space and resources, may need to come through political acknowledgement and allocation. Indeed Sakti (2013, 449) demonstrates the healing importance of "financial assistance from the Timorese government in order to deliver payment for delayed mortuary rituals" necessary, above and beyond material necessity, to restore reciprocal lines of exchange and obligation that constitute East Timorese society and the ongoing "flow of life."

Successful intervention are likely those that combine the structural with those that facilitate agency. Silove's (1999, 2013) ADAPT framework (*Adaptation and Development After Persecution and Trauma*) positions the establishment of social justice alongside "systems that support conditions of security and safety, the integrity of family and community bonds, the capacity to pursue roles and identities, and the ability to engage in practices that confer existential meaning (political, religious, spiritual, social, cultural)" (Le Touze et al. 2005, 198) as necessary foundations for individual and communal recovery from trauma. As should be clear from our model, we would see no reason at all why such principles should not apply to cases of psychosis, and we would expect overall prevalence and relapse rates to decrease under such ideal circumstances.

Where more psychosis-specific interventions are needed, besides the dilemma of possible judicious use of medication (ideally framed as a "palliative" coping measure to ensure the task of attending to wider maintaining causes is not lost cf. Moncrieff 2013) we should surely aim for interventions that respect and enrich existing cultural ways of being and coping. Approaches based on the Finnish *Open Dialogue* social network model might be argued to particularly suitable for exploring both "mundane" (relating to histories of colonial occupation and violence) and symbolic dimensions of psychotic behaviour in a culturally sensitive manner (Seikkula et al. 2001; see Sects. 5.1.3 and 5.2.3). Open Dialogue aims, through facilitated conversation, to empower individuals and family networks to make decisions while also, being grounded in the epistemology of family therapy, being able to reflect on possible "functional" aspects of illness. Similarly the burgeoning interest in indirect or even direct dialogue with "psychotic" voices (Corstens et al. 2012; Hayward et al. 2009; Sect. 5.1.2) may mirror the relational approaches traditionally employed in ritual negotiations with spiritual entities such as *rai nain* carrying possibilities of mutual enrichment. As we have argued narrative is the thread that weaves between agentic and deterministic positions and experience, and in the context of a formal ritualised space, where more emotional communication might be permitted (cf. Sakti 2013), some adaption of Narrative Exposure Therapy for trauma (Buda et al. 2005) might also be acceptable.

Perhaps this irreconcilable separation of the deterministic from the agentic is exactly why one cultural consultant discussed earlier was indeed insistent that the political and the sacred are separate domains that cannot be conflated—while the political and the sacred might ultimately belong to an original unity (see Sect. 2.3.4, incl. Footnote 16), thinking about such spheres of action and experience, demands they are treated separately.[27]

References

Aaltonen, Jukka, and Viljo Räkköläinen. 1994. The shared image guiding the treatment process: A precondition for integration of the treatment of schizophrenia. *The British Journal of Psychiatry* 164(Suppl 23): 97–102.

Aaltonen, J., J. Seikkula, and K. Lehtinen. 2011. The comprehensive open-dialogue approach in Western Lapland: I. The incidence of non-affective psychosis and prodromal states. *Psychosis* 3(3): 179–191.

Alanen, Yrjö O. 1997. *Schizophrenia: Its origins and need-adapted treatment*. London: Karnac Books.

Aleman, Andre, Rene S. Kahn, and Jean-Paul Selten. 2003. Sex differences in the risk of schizophrenia: Evidence from meta-analysis. *Archives of General Psychiatry* 60(6): 565–571. doi:10.1001/archpsyc.60.6.565.

Allen, John S. 1997. At issue: Are traditional societies schizophrenogenic? *Schizophrenia Bulletin* 23(3): 357.

American Psychiatric Association (APA). 2013. *Diagnostic and Statistical Manual of Mental Disorders, Fifth Edition*, 5th ed. Washington, DC: Author.

Angermeyer, Matthias C., Anita Holzinger, Mauro G. Carta, and Georg Schomerus. 2011. Biogenetic explanations and public acceptance of mental illness: Systematic review of population studies. *The British Journal of Psychiatry* 199(5): 367–372. doi:10.1192/bjp.bp.110.085563.

[27]In essence politics concerns worldly power, and the seeking of supposedly "rational" solutions that impact on the material world. The sacred is more concerned with relationships and meaning (although the associated practice of magic might claim to change the material world, to the detached observer it is clear that it is more about the manipulation of meaning). Of course political aims begin with human agency, are often inextricably tied to relationships and might sometimes be accused of the manipulation of meaning ("spin")—but as ideal types the distinction holds.

Arana, George W. 2000. an overview of side effects caused by typical antipsychotics. *Journal of Clinical Psychiatry* 61(Suppl 8): 5–11.

Atchison, Michael, and A.C. McFarlane. 1994. A review of dissociation and dissociative disorders. *Australian and New Zealand Journal of Psychiatry* 28(4): 591–599.

Barrett, Robert J. 2004. 'Kurt Schneider in Borneo: Do first rank symptoms apply to the Iban?' In *Schizophrenia, culture, and subjectivity: The edge of experience*, eds. Janis Hunter Jenkins and Robert J. Barrett, 87–109. Cambridge, UK: Cambridge University Press.

Bell, Morris D., Paul H. Lysaker, and Robert M. Milstein. 1996. Clinical benefits of paid work activity in schizophrenia. *Schizophrenia Bulletin* 22(1): 51.

Belsky, J., C. Jonassaint, M. Pluess, M. Stanton, B. Brummett, and R. Williams. 2009. Vulnerability genes or plasticity genes. *Molecular Psychiatry* 14(8): 746–754.

Berrios, German E. 2014. History and epistemology of psychopathology. In *Philosophical issues in psychiatry III: The nature and sources of historical change*, eds. Kenneth S. Kendler, and Josef Parnas, 30–50. Oxford, UK: Oxford University Press. EPUB file.

Boddy, J. 1988. Spirits and selves in Northern Sudan: The cultural therapeutics of possession and trance. *American Ethnologist* 15(1): 4–27.

Boddy, J. 1994. Spirit possession revisited: Beyond instrumentality. *Annual Review of Anthropology* 23: 407–434.

Bovensiepen, Judith. 2009. Spiritual landscapes of life and death in the central highlands of East Timor. *Anthropological Forum* 19: 323–338.

Boydell, Dr J., Prof J. van Os, Dr K. McKenzie, and Prof R.M. Murray. 2004. The association of inequality with the incidence of schizophrenia. *Social Psychiatry and Psychiatric Epidemiology* 39(8): 597–599. doi:10.1007/s00127-004-0789-6.

Brand, Bethany L., Catherine C. Classen, Scot W. McNary, and Parin Zaveri. 2009. A review of dissociative disorders treatment studies. *The Journal of Nervous and Mental Disease* 197(9): 646–654.

Brand, Bethany L., Amie C. Myrick, Richard J. Loewenstein, Catherine C. Classen, Ruth Lanius, Scot W. McNary, Clare Pain, and Frank W. Putnam. 2012. A survey of practices and recommended treatment interventions among expert therapists treating patients with dissociative identity disorder and dissociative disorder not otherwise specified. *Psychological Trauma: Theory, Research, Practice, and Policy* 4(5): 490–500. doi:10.1037/a0026487.

Buda, Béla, M. Schauer, F. Neuner, and T. Elbert. 2005. Narrative exposure therapy. A short-term intervention for traumatic stress disorders after war, terror, or torture. *Crisis: The Journal of Crisis Intervention and Suicide Prevention* 26(4): 194–95. doi:10.1027/0227-5910.26.4.194b.

Burns, Jan. 1992. Mad or just plain bad? Gender and the work of forensic clinical psychologists. In *Gender issues in clinical psychology*, eds. Jane M. Ussher and Paula Nicolson, 106–128. London: Routledge.

Burns, Jonathan K., and Tonya Esterhuizen. 2008. Poverty, inequality and the treated incidence of first-episode psychosis. *Social Psychiatry and Psychiatric Epidemiology* 43(4): 331–335. doi:10.1007/s00127-008-0308-2.

Castagnini, Augusto C. 2010. Wimmer's concept of psychogenic psychosis revisited. *History of Psychiatry* 21(1): 54–66. doi:10.1177/0957154X09338086.

Castagnini, Augusto, and German E. Berrios. 2011. The relationship of acute transient psychoses and schizophrenia. In *Handbook of schizophrenia spectrum disorders*, vol. II, ed. Michael Ritsner, 367–387. Dordrecht: Springer.

Chakrabarti, Subho. 2011. Family interventions in schizophrenia: Issues of relevance for Asian countries. *World Journal of Psychiatry* 1(1): 4–7. doi:10.5498/wjp.v1.i1.4.

Cheng, Andrew T.A. 2002. Expressed emotion: A cross-culturally valid concept? *The British Journal of Psychiatry* 181(6): 466–467.

Climent, Carlos E., and Robert Plutchik. 1977. Lunar madness: An empirical study. *Comprehensive Psychiatry* 18(4): 369–374. doi:10.1016/0010-440X(77)90009-8.

Corin, Ellen, Thara Rangaswami, and Padmavati Ramachandran. 2004. Living through a staggering world: The play of signifiers in early psychosis in South India. In *Schizophrenia,*

culture, and subjectivity: The edge of experience, eds. Janis Hunter Jenkins and Robert J. Barrett, 110–145. Cambridge, UK: Cambridge University Press.
Corrigan, Patrick W. 2007. How clinical diagnosis might exacerbate the stigma of mental illness. *Social Work* 52(1): 31–39. doi:10.1093/sw/52.1.31.
Corstens, Dirk, Eleanor Longden, and Rufus May. 2012. Talking with voices: Exploring what is expressed by the voices people hear. *Psychosis* 4(2): 95–104. doi:10.1080/17522439.2011.571705.
Cox, Rochelle E., and Amanda J. Barnier. 2010. Hypnotic illusions and clinical delusions: Hypnosis as a research method. *Cognitive Neuropsychiatry* 15(1–3): 202–232. doi:10.1080/13546800903319884.
de Haan, Lieuwe, Don H. Linszen, Marie E. Lenior, Evelyne Dodertein de Win, and Rob Gorsira. 2003. Duration of untreated psychosis and outcome of schizophrenia: Delay in intensive psychosocial treatment versus delay in treatment with antipsychotic medication. *Schizophrenia Bulletin* 29(2): 341–348.
DelVecchio Good, Mary-Jo. 2013. Perspectives on trauma and healing from anthropology and social and affective neuroscience. *Transcultural Psychiatry* 50(5): 744–52. doi:10.1177/1363461513508174.
Eigen, Michael. 2004. *The psychotic core*. London: Karnac Books.
Falicov, Celia Jaes. 1995. Training to think culturally: A multidimensional comparative framework. *Family Process* 34(4): 373–388. doi:10.1111/j.1545-5300.1995.00373.x.
Fonagy, Peter, Gyorgy Gergely, Elliot Jurist, and Mary Target. 2002. *Affect regulation, mentalization, and the development of the self*. New York: Other Press.
Frosh, Stephen. 2006. *For and against psychoanalysis*. London: Routledge.
Gainer, Karen. 1994. Dissociation and schizophrenia: An historical review of conceptual development and relevant treatment approaches. *Dissociation* 7(4): 261–271.
Geertz, C. 1973. *The interpretation of cultures*. New York: HarperCollins Basic Books.
Geertz, Clifford. 1984. "From the Native's Point of View": On the nature of anthropological understanding. In *Culture theory: Essays on mind, self and emotion*, eds. Richard A. Shweder and Robert A. LeVine, 123–136. Cambridge: Cambridge University Press.
Gergely, György, and John S. Watson. 1999. Early socio-emotional development: Contingency perception and the social-biofeedback model. In *Early Social Cognition: Understanding Others in the First Months of Life*, ed. Philippe Rochat, 101–36. Hillsdale, NJ: Lawrence Erlbaum Associates.
Guinness, E.A. 1992a. Brief reactive psychosis and the major functional psychoses: Descriptive case studies in Africa. *The British Journal of Psychiatry. Supplement*, no. 16 (April): 24–41.
Guinness, E.A. 1992b. Relationship between the neuroses and brief reactive psychosis: Descriptive case studies in Africa. *The British Journal of Psychiatry. Supplement*, no. 16 (April): 12–23.
Haigh, Rex. 2012. The philosophy of greencare: Why it matters for our mental health. *Mental Health and Social Inclusion* 16(3): 127–134. doi:10.1108/20428301211255400.
Halliburton, Murphy. 2009. *Mudpacks and Prozac: Experiencing ayurvedic, biomedical, and religious healing*. Left Coast Press.
Harrison, S. 2004. Emotional climates: Ritual, seasonality and affective disorders. *Journal of the Royal Anthropological Institute* 10(3): 583–603.
Harrow, Martin, and Thomas H. Jobe. 2007. Factors involved in outcome and recovery in schizophrenia patients not on antipsychotic medications: A 15-year multifollow-up study. *The Journal of Nervous and Mental Disease* 195(5): 406–414. doi:10.1097/01.nmd.0000253783.32338.6e.
Hashemi, Amtul H., and Raymond Cochrane. 1999. Expressed emotion and schizophrenia: A review of studies across cultures. *International Review of Psychiatry* 11(2–3): 219–224. doi:10.1080/09540269974401.
Hayward, Mark, Jo Overton, Theresa Dorey, and Joanna Denney. 2009. Relating therapy for people who hear voices: A case series. *Clinical Psychology & Psychotherapy* 16(3): 216–227. doi:10.1002/cpp.615.

Hicks, David. 1984. *A maternal religion: The role of women in Tetum Myth and Ritual*. Monograph Series of Southeast Asia. Northern Illinois University, Center for Southeast Asian Studies.

Hicks, David. 2004. *Tetum ghosts & kin: Fertility and gender in East Timor*, 2nd ed. Waveland Pr Inc.

Hollan, D. 2013. Coping in plain sight: Work as a local response to event-related emotional distress in contemporary U.S. Society. *Transcultural Psychiatry* 50(5): 726–743. doi:10.1177/1363461513488077.

Hopper, Kim. 1991. Some old questions for the new cross-cultural psychiatry. *Medical Anthropology Quarterly*, New Series, 5(4): 299–330.

Hopper, Kim. 2004. Interrogating the meaning of "culture" in the WHO international studies of schizophrenia. In *Schizophrenia, culture, and subjectivity: The edge of experience*, eds. Janis Hunter Jenkins and Robert J. Barrett, 62–86. Cambridge, UK: Cambridge University Press.

Hopper, Kim. 2008. Outcomes elsewhere: Course of psychosis in "Other Cultures". In *Society and psychosis*, eds. Craig Morgan, Kwame McKenzie and Paul Fearon, 198–216. Cambridge: Cambridge University Press.

Hopper, Kim, Glynn Harrison, Aleksandar Janca, and Norman Sartorius, eds. 2007. *Recovery from schizophrenia: An international perspective : A report from the WHO Collaborative Project, the international study of schizophrenia*. Oxford: Oxford University Press.

Hopper, K., J. Wanderling, and P. Narayanan. 2007b. To have and to hold: A cross-cultural inquiry into marital prospects after psychosis. *Global Public Health* 2(3): 257–280. doi:10.1080/17441690600855778.

Jackson, Murray. 2001. *Weathering storms: Psychotherapy for psychosis*. Karnac Books.

Jadhav, Sushrut. 2007. Dhis and Dhāt: Evidence of semen retention syndrome amongst White Britons. *Anthropology & Medicine* 14(3): 229–239. doi:10.1080/13648470701772770.

Jadhav, Sushrut, Roland Littlewood, Andrew G. Ryder, Ajita Chakraborty, Sumeet Jain, and Maan Barua. 2007. Stigmatization of severe mental illness in India: Against the simple industrialization hypothesis. *Indian Journal of Psychiatry* 49(3): 189–194. doi:10.4103/0019-5545.37320.

Jaynes, Julian. 2000. *The origin of consciousness in the breakdown of the bicameral mind*. Houghton Mifflin Harcourt.

Jenkins, J.H. 1988. Ethnopsychiatric interpretations of schizophrenic illness: The problem of nervios within Mexican-American families. *Culture, Medicine and Psychiatry* 12(3): 301–329.

Jenkins, Janis Hunter. 1991. Anthropology, expressed emotion, and schizophrenia. *Ethos* 19(4): 387–431.

Jilek, W.G., and L. Jilek-Aall. 1970. Transient psychoses in Africans. *Psychopathology* 3(6): 337–364.

Joseph, Jay. 2006. *The missing gene: Psychiatry, heredity, and the fruitless search for genes*. Algora Pub.

Kirkbride, J.B., P.B. Jones, S. Ullrich, and J.W. Coid. 2014. Social deprivation, inequality, and the neighborhood-level incidence of psychotic syndromes in East London. *Schizophrenia Bulletin* 40(1): 169–180. doi:10.1093/schbul/sbs151.

Kirmayer, Laurence J. 1996. Confusion of the senses: Implications of ethnocultural variations in somatoform and dissociative disorders for PTSD. In *Ethnocultural aspects of posttraumatic stress disorder: Issues, research, and clinical applications*, eds. Anthony J. Marsella, Matthew J. Friedman, Ellen T. Gerrity, and Raymond M. Scurfield, 131–163. Washington, DC: American Psychological Association.

Kirmayer, Laurence J. 2011. Defining and delimiting trauma-related dissociation: A view from cultural psychiatry. *Journal of Trauma & Dissociation* 12(4): 465–468. doi:10.1080/15299732.2011.570235.

Kirmayer, Laurence J. 1994. Pacing the void: Social and cultural dimensions of dissociation. In *Dissociation: Culture, mind, and body*, ed. David Spiegel, 91–122.

Kirmayer, Laurence J., and Ellen Corin. 1998. Inside knowledge: Cultural constructions of insight in psychosis. In *Insight and psychosis*, eds. Xavier Francisco Amador and Anthony S. David, 193–220. New York: Oxford University Press.

Laddis, Andreas, and Paul F. Dell. 2012. Dissociation and psychosis in dissociative identity disorder and schizophrenia. *Journal of Trauma & Dissociation* 13(4): 397–413. doi:10.1080/15299732.2012.664967.

Last, M. 2000. Healing the social wounds of war. *Medicine, Conflict, and Survival* 16(4): 370–382.

Le Touze, D., D. Silove, and A. Zwi. 2005. Can there be healing without justice? Lessons from the commission for reception, truth and reconciliation in East Timor. *Intervention* 3(3): 192–202.

Leeson, Verity C., Thomas R.E. Barnes, Masuma Harrison, Elizabeth Matheson, Isobel Harrison, Stanley H. Mutsatsa, Maria A. Ron, and Eileen M. Joyce. 2010. The relationship between IQ, memory, executive function, and processing speed in recent-onset psychosis: 1-year stability and clinical outcome. *Schizophrenia Bulletin* 36(2): 400–409. doi:10.1093/schbul/sbn100.

Leff, Julian, Geoffrey Williams, Mark Huckvale, Maurice Arbuthnot, and Alex P. Leff. 2013a. Avatar therapy for persecutory auditory hallucinations: What is it and how does it work? *Psychosis*, no. ahead-of-print: 1–11.

Leff, Julian, G. Williams, M.A. Huckvale, M. Arbuthnot, and A.P. Leff. 2013b. Computer-assisted therapy for medication-resistant auditory hallucinations: Proof-of-concept study. *The British Journal of Psychiatry* 202(6): 428–433. doi:10.1192/bjp.bp.112.124883.

Lilienfeld, S.O., and L. Marino. 1995. Mental disorder as a Roschian concept: A critique of Wakefield's "Harmful Dysfunction" analysis. *Journal of Abnormal Psychology* 104(3): 411–420.

Littlewood, Roland. 1996. *Reason and necessity in the specification of the multiple self.* Royal Anthropological Institute.

Littlewood, Roland, and Maurice Lipsedge. 1987. The butterfly and the serpent: Culture, psychopathology and biomedicine. *Culture, Medicine and Psychiatry* 11(3): 289–335.

Littlewood, Roland, and Simon Dein. 2013. Did christianity lead to schizophrenia? Psychosis, psychology and self reference. *Transcultural Psychiatry* 50(3): 397–420. doi:10.1177/1363461513489681.

Littlewood, Roland, Sushrut Jadhav, and Andrew G. Ryder. 2007. A cross-national study of the stigmatization of severe psychiatric illness: Historical review, methodological considerations and development of the questionnaire. *Transcultural Psychiatry* 44(2): 171–202. doi:10.1177/1363461507077720.

London, Nathaniel J. 1973. An essay on psychoanalytic theory: Two theories of schizophrenia: I. review and critical assessment of the development of the two theories. *The International Journal of Psychoanalysis*. http://psycnet.apa.org/psycinfo/1975-03319-001.

Lucas, R.H., and R.J. Barrett. 1995. Interpreting culture and psychopathology: Primitivist themes in cross-cultural debate. *Culture, Medicine and Psychiatry* 19(3): 287–326.

Luhrmann, T.M. 2007. Social defeat and the culture of chronicity: Or, why schizophrenia does so well over there and so badly here. *Culture, Medicine and Psychiatry* 31(2): 135–172. doi:10.1007/s11013-007-9049-z.

Luhrmann, T.M. 2013. Making God real and making God good: Some mechanisms through which prayer may contribute to healing. *Transcultural Psychiatry* 50(5): 707–725. doi:10.1177/1363461513487670.

Luhrmann, T.M., R. Padmavati, H. Tharoor, and A. Osei. 2015. Differences in voice-hearing experiences of people with psychosis in the USA, India and Ghana: Interview-based study. *The British Journal of Psychiatry* 206(1): 41–44. doi:10.1192/bjp.bp.113.139048.

Marneros, Andreas, and Frank Pillmann. 2004. *Acute and transient psychoses*. Cambridge: Cambridge University Press.

McCrae, Niall. 2011. *The Moon and madness*. EPUB file: Andrews UK Limited.

McGlashan, Thomas H., Steven T. Levy, and William T. Carpenter. 1975. Integration and sealing over: Clinically distinct recovery styles from schizophrenia. *Archives of General Psychiatry* 32 (10): 1269–1272. doi:10.1001/archpsyc.1975.01760280067006.

McGruder, Juli H. 2004. Madness in Zanzibar: An exploration of lived experience. In *Schizophrenia, culture, and subjectivity: The edge of experience*, eds. by Janis Hunter Jenkins and Robert J. Barrett, 255–381. Cambridge, UK: Cambridge University Press.

McLean, Duncan, Rangaswamy Thara, Sujit John, Robert Barrett, Peter Loa, John McGrath, and Bryan Mowry. 2014. DSM-IV "Criterion A" schizophrenia symptoms across ethnically different populations: Evidence for differing psychotic symptom content or structural organization? *Culture, Medicine and Psychiatry* 38(3): 408–426. doi:10.1007/s11013-014-9385-8.

McWilliam, Andrew, and Elizabeth G. Traube. 2011. Introduction. In *Land and life in Timor-Leste: Ethnographic essays*, eds. Andrew McWilliam, and Elizabeth G. Traube. Canberra, ACT, Australia: ANU E Press. (EPUB file).

Moncrieff, Joanna. 2013. *The bitterest pills: The troubling story of antipsychotic drugs*. London: Palgrave Macmillan.

Morrison, Anthony P., Douglas Turkington, Melissa Pyle, Helen Spencer, Alison Brabban, Graham Dunn, Tom Christodoulides, et al. 2014. Cognitive therapy for people with schizophrenia spectrum disorders not taking antipsychotic drugs: A single-blind randomised controlled trial. *The Lancet, February*. doi:10.1016/S0140-6736(13)62246-1.

Moskowitz, Andrew. 2012. Commentary on "Dissociation and Psychosis in Dissociative Identity Disorder and Schizophrenia" (Laddis & Dell). *Journal of Trauma & Dissociation* 13(4): 414–417. doi:10.1080/15299732.2011.621017.

Moskowitz, Andrew. 2008. Association and dissociation in the historical concept of schizophrenia. In *Psychosis, trauma and dissociation: Emerging perspectives on severe psychopathology*, eds. Andrew Moskowitz, Ingo Schäfer, and Martin Justin Dorahy, 1475–1903. Chichester, West Sussex. UK: Wiley-Blackwell. Kindle file.

Moskowitz, Andrew, Suzanne Barker-Collo, and Lynsey Ellson. 2005. Replication of dissociation-psychosis link in New Zealand students and inmates. *The Journal of Nervous and Mental Disease* 193(11): 722–727.

Motjabai, Ramin, Ezra Susser, and Vijoy Varma. 2000. Duration of remitting psychoses with acute onset: Implications for ICD-10. *The British Journal of Psychiatry* 176(6): 576–580. doi:10.1192/bjp.176.6.576.

Murphy, H.B.M. 1968. Cultural factors in the genesis of schizophrenia. *Journal of Psychiatric Research* 6(November): 137–153. doi:10.1016/0022-3956(68)90013-7.

Murphy, H.B.M., and G. Vega. 1982. Schizophrenia and religious affiliation in Northern Ireland. *Psychological Medicine* 12(03): 595–605. doi:10.1017/S0033291700055707.

Myers, Neely Laurenzo. 2010. Culture, stress and recovery from schizophrenia: Lessons from the field for global mental health. *Culture, Medicine and Psychiatry* 34(3): 500–528. doi:10.1007/s11013-010-9186-7.

Myers, Neely Laurenzo. 2011. Update: schizophrenia across cultures. *Current Psychiatry Reports* 13(4): 305–311. doi:10.1007/s11920-011-0208-0.

Nasser, Elizabeth H., Natalie Walders, and Janis H. Jenkins. 2002. The experience of schizophrenia: What's gender got to do with it? A critical review of the current status of research on schizophrenia. *Schizophrenia Bulletin* 28(2): 351.

Nijenhuis, Ellert R.S., and Onno van der Hart. 2011. Dissociation in trauma: A new definition and comparison with previous formulations. *Journal of Trauma & Dissociation* 12(4): 416–445. doi:10.1080/15299732.2011.570592.

Nordgaard, Julie, Sidse M. Arnfred, Peter Handest, and Josef Parnas. 2008. The diagnostic status of first-rank symptoms. *Schizophrenia Bulletin* 34(1): 137–154. doi:10.1093/schbul/sbm044.

Obeyesekere. 1984. *Medusa's hair: An essay on personal symbols and religious experience*. Chicago: University of Chicago Press (Kindle file).

Oda, Ana Maria G. Raimundo, Claudio Eduardo M. Banzato, and Paulo Dalgalarrondo. 2005. Some origins of cross-cultural psychiatry. *History of Psychiatry* 16(2): 155–169.

Ortner, Sherry B. 1973. On key symbols. *American Anthropologist*, New Series, 75(5): 1338–1346. doi:10.2307/674036.

Pearce, W. Barnett. 2007. *Making social worlds: A communication perspective*. Oxford, UK: Blackwell.

Perry, B.D., R.A. Pollard, T.L. Blakley, W.L. Baker, and D. Vigilante. 1995. Childhood trauma, the neurobiology of adaptation, and "use-Dependent" development of the brain: How "states" become "traits". *Infant Mental Health Journal* 16(4): 271–291.

Pestalozzi, Julia. 2003. The symbolic and concrete: Psychotic adolescents in psychoanalytic psychotherapy. *The International Journal of Psychoanalysis* 84(3): 733–753. doi:10.1516/G6AC-WEHN-EBWM-5VD9.

Piccinelli, Marco, and Francesca Gomez Homen. 1997. *Gender differences in the epidemiology of affective disorders and schizophrenia*. Geneva: Division of Mental Health and Prevention of Substance Abuse, World Health Organization. http://apps.who.int/iris/handle/10665/63505.

Pillmann, F., A. Haring, S. Balzuweit, R. Blöink, and A. Marneros. 2000. Concordance of acute and transient psychoses and cycloid psychoses. *Psychopathology* 34(6): 305–311.

Pillmann, F., and A. Marneros. 2003. Brief and acute psychoses: The development of concepts. *History of Psychiatry* 14(2): 161–177. doi:10.1177/0957154X030142002.

Pillmann, F., A. Haring, S. Balzuweit, R. Blöink, and A. Marneros. 2002. The concordance of ICD-10 acute and transient psychosis and DSM-IV brief psychotic disorder. *Psychological Medicine* 32(3): 525–533.

Pillmann, Frank, Annette Haring, Sabine Balzuweit, Raffaela Blöink, and Andreas Marneros. 2003. Bouffée Délirante and ICD-10 acute and transient psychoses: A comparative study. *The Australian and New Zealand Journal of Psychiatry* 37(3): 327–333.

Read, U. 2012. "I Want the One That Will Heal Me Completely so It Won't Come Back Again": The limits of antipsychotic medication in Rural Ghana. *Transcultural Psychiatry* 49(3–4): 438–460. doi:10.1177/1363461512447070.

Read, John, Paul Fink, Thom Rudegeair, Vincent Felitti, and Charles Whitfield. 2008. Child maltreatment and psychosis: A return to a genuinely integrated bio-psycho-social model. *Clinical Schizophrenia & Related Psychoses* 2(3): 235–254. doi:10.3371/CSRP.2.3.5.

Read, John, Roar Fosse, Andrew Moskowitz, and Bruce Perry. 2014. The traumagenic neurodevelopmental model of psychosis revisited. *Neuropsychiatry* 4(1): 65–79. doi:10.2217/npy.13.89.

Regier, D.A., W.E. Narrow, E.A. Kuhl, and D.J. Kupfer. 2009. The conceptual development of DSM-V. *American Journal of Psychiatry* 166(6): 645.

Rosenbaum, Milton. 1980. The role of the term schizophrenia in the decline of diagnoses of multiple personality. *Archives of General Psychiatry* 37(12): 1383–1385. doi:10.1001/archpsyc.1980.01780250069008.

Ross, Colin A. 2006. *The trauma model: A solution to the problem of comorbidity in psychiatry*. Richardson, TX: Manitou Communications.

Ross, Colin A. 2014. Problems with the psychosis section of DSM-5. *Psychosis* 6(3): 235–241. doi:10.1080/17522439.2013.839736.

Ross, Colin A. 2008. Dissociative schizophrenia. In *Psychosis, trauma and dissociation: Emerging perspectives on severe psychopathology*, eds. Andrew Moskowitz, Ingo Schäfer, and Martin Justin Dorahy, 8433–8801. Chichester, West Sussex. UK: Wiley-Blackwell (Kindle file).

Ross, C.A., S.D. Miller, P. Reagor, L. Bjornson, G.A. Fraser, and G. Anderson. 1990. Schneiderian symptoms in multiple personality disorder and schizophrenia. *Comprehensive Psychiatry* 31(2): 111–118.

Rubio, Jose M., Julio Sanjuán, Ludwing Flórez-Salamanca, and Manuel J. Cuesta. 2012. Examining the course of hallucinatory experiences in children and adolescents: A systematic review. *Schizophrenia Research* 138(2–3): 248–254. doi:10.1016/j.schres.2012.03.012.

Sakti, Victoria Kumala. 2013. "Thinking Too Much": Tracing local patterns of emotional distress after mass violence in Timor-Leste. *The Asia Pacific Journal of Anthropology* 14(5): 438–454. doi:10.1080/14442213.2013.826733.

Sass, Louis A. 1992. *Madness and modernism: Insanity in the light of modern art, literature, and thought*. New York, NY.: Basic Books.

Sass, Louis A. 2001. Self and world in schizophrenia: Three classic approaches. *Philosophy, Psychiatry, & Psychology* 8(4): 251–270. doi:10.1353/ppp.2002.0026.

Sass, Louis A. 1995. *The paradoxes of delusion: Wittgenstein, Schreber, and the schizophrenic mind*. Cornell University Press.

Sass, Louis A., and Josef Parnas. 2003. Schizophrenia, consciousness, and the self. *Schizophrenia Bulletin* 29(3): 427–444.

Saha, Sukanta, David Chant, Joy Welham, and John McGrath. 2005. A systematic review of the prevalence of schizophrenia. *PLoS Medicine* 2(5): e141. doi:10.1371/journal.pmed.0020141.

Scharfetter, Christian. 2008. Ego-fragmentation in schizophrenia: A severe dissociation of self-experience. In *Psychosis, trauma and dissociation: Emerging perspectives on severe psychopathology*, eds. Andrew Moskowitz, Ingo Schäfer, and Martin Justin Dorahy, 1925–2270. Chichester, West Sussex. UK: Wiley-Blackwell. Kindle file.

Scheff, T.J. 1970. Schizophrenia as ideology. *Schizophrenia Bulletin* 1(2): 15–19. doi:10.1093/schbul/1.2.15.

Scheper-Hughes, Nancy. 2001. *Saints, scholars and schizophrenics: Mental illness in Rural Ireland*. Twentieth anniversary ed, updated and expanded edition. Berkeley: University of California Press.

Searles, H.F. 1958. The schizophrenic's vulnerability to the therapist's unconscious processes. *The Journal of Nervous and Mental Disease* 127(3): 247–262.

Seikkula, J., B. Alakare, and J. Aaltonen. 2001. Open Dialogue in psychosis I: An introduction and case illustration. *Journal of Constructivist Psychology* 14(4): 247–265.

Seikkula, J., B. Alakare, and J. Aaltonen. 2011. The comprehensive open-dialogue approach in Western Lapland: II. Long-term stability of acute psychosis outcomes in advanced community care. *Psychosis* 3(3): 192–204.

Seligman, Rebecca. 2005. Distress, dissociation, and embodied experience: Reconsidering the pathways to mediumship and mental health. *Ethos* 33(1): 71–99.

Shaver, Phillip R., and R. Chris Fraley. 2008. Attachment, loss and grief: Bowlby's views and current controversies. In *Handbook of attachment*, 2nd ed., eds. Jude Cassidy and Phillip R. Shaver, 48–77. New York, NY: Guilford Press.

Silove, D. 1999. The psychosocial effects of torture, mass human rights violations, and refugee trauma: Toward an integrated conceptual framework. *The Journal of Nervous and Mental Disease* 187(4): 200.

Silove, Derrick. 2005. The best immediate therapy for acute stress is social. *Bulletin of the World Health Organization* 83(1): 75–76.

Silove, Derrick. 2013. The ADAPT model: A conceptual framework for mental health and psychosocial programming in post conflict settings. *Intervention* 11(3). http://journals.lww.com/interventionjnl/Fulltext/2013/11000/The_ADAPT_model___a_conceptual_framework_for.2.aspx.

Silove, Derrick, Catherine Robina Bateman, Robert T. Brooks, C. Amaral Zulmira Fonseca, Zachary Steel, James Rodger, Ian Soosay, Greg Fox, Vikram Patel, and Adrian Bauman. 2008. Estimating clinically relevant mental disorders in a rural and an urban setting in postconflict Timor Leste. *Archives of General Psychiatry* 65(10): 1205–1212. doi:10.1001/archpsyc.65.10.1205.

Singh, Swaran P. 2011. Acute and transient psychotic disorders. In *Current themes in psychiatry in theory and practice*, eds. Niruj Agrawal, Jim Bolton, and Raghunandan Gaind, 77–98. London: Palgrave Macmillan.

Singh, Swaran P., Tom Burns, Shazad Amin, Peter B. Jones, and Glynn Harrison. 2004. Acute and transient psychotic disorders: Precursors, epidemiology, course and outcome. *The British Journal of Psychiatry* 185(6): 452–459. doi:10.1192/bjp.185.6.452.

Singh, S.P., K. Harley, and K. Suhail. 2013. Cultural specificity of emotional overinvolvement: A systematic review. *Schizophrenia Bulletin* 39(2): 449–463. doi:10.1093/schbul/sbr170.

Stern, Daniel N. 2003. Introduction to the paperback edition. In *The interpersonal world of the infant: A view from psychoanalysis and developmental psychology*, Paperback edition, xi–xxxix. London: Karnac Books.

Stevens, Janice. 1987. Brief psychoses: Do they contribute to the good prognosis and equal prevalence of schizophrenia in developing countries? *The British Journal of Psychiatry* 151(3): 393–396.
Subandi, M.A. 2011. Family expressed emotion in a Javanese cultural context. *Culture, Medicine and Psychiatry* 35(3): 331–346. doi:10.1007/s11013-011-9220-4.
Susser, Ezra, and Joseph Wanderling. 1994. Epidemiology of nonaffective acute remitting psychosis vs schizophrenia: Sex and sociocultural setting. *Archives of General Psychiatry* 51 (4): 294–301. doi:10.1001/archpsyc.1994.03950040038005.
Teicher, M.H., S.L. Andersen, A. Polcari, C.M. Anderson, C.P. Navalta, and D.M. Kim. 2003. The neurobiological consequences of early stress and childhood maltreatment. *Neuroscience and Biobehavioral Reviews* 27(1–2): 33–44.
Thompson, Andrew, Sarah Sullivan, Glyn Lewis, Stanley Zammit, Jon Heron, Jeremy Horwood, Kate Thomas, et al. 2011. Association between locus of control in childhood and psychotic symptoms in early adolescence: Results from a large birth cohort. *Cognitive Neuropsychiatry* 16(5): 385–402. doi:10.1080/13546805.2010.546077.
Tienari, P., L.C. Wynne, J. Moring, I. Lahti, M. Naarala, A. Sorri, K.E. Wahlberg, O. Saarento, M. Seitamaa, and M. Kaleva. 1994. The finnish adoptive family study of schizophrenia. Implications for family research. *The British Journal of Psychiatry. Supplement*, no. 23(April): 20–26.
Toome, Emily. 2012. "Filling Wounds with Salt": The pathologisation of trauma in Timor-Leste. In *Local-global*, traversing customary community and modern nation-formation in Timor-Leste, ed. Damian Grenfell, vol. 11, 24–30.
Tranulis, Constantin, Lawrence Park, Laura Delano, and Byron Good. 2009. Early intervention in psychosis: A case study on normal and pathological. *Culture, Medicine and Psychiatry* 33(4): 608–622. doi:10.1007/s11013-009-9150-6.
Traube, Elizabeth G. 1986. *Cosmology and social life: Ritual exchange among the Mambai of East Timor*. Chicago: University of Chicago Press.
Traube, Elizabeth G. 2007. Unpaid wages: local narratives and the imagination of the nation. *The Asia Pacific Journal of Anthropology* 8(1): 9–25. doi:10.1080/14442210601161724.
Traube, Elizabeth G. 2011. Painting the Flag. In *Land and life in Timor-Leste: Ethnographic essays*, eds. Andrew McWilliam, and Elizabeth G. Traube, 117–140. Canberra, ACT, Australia: ANU E Press. EPUB file
Turner, Victor. 1967. *The forest of symbols*. London: Cornell University Press.
Üçok, Alp, and Wolfgang Gaebel. 2008. Side effects of atypical antipsychotics: A brief overview. *World Psychiatry* 7(1): 58–62.
Ugarte, Eduardo. 1992. Running Amok: The "demoniacal Impulse". *Asian Studies Review* 16(1): 182–189.
van der Geest, Sjaak, and Susan Reynolds Whyte. 1989. The charm of medicines: Metaphors and metonyms. *Medical Anthropology Quarterly*, New Series, 3(4): 345–367.
van der Hart, Onno, Ellert Nijenhuis, Kathy Steele, and Daniel Brown. 2004. Trauma-related dissociation: Conceptual clarity lost and found. *Australian and New Zealand Journal of Psychiatry* 38(11–12): 906–914. doi:10.1111/j.1440-1614.2004.01480.x.
Van der Kolk, Bessel A., David Pelcovitz, Susan Roth, F.S. Mandel, Alexander McFarlane, and Judith L. Herman. 1996. Dissociation, somatization, and affect dysregulation: The complexity of adaptation to trauma. *American Journal of Psychiatry* 153(7): 83–93.
Walsh, Roger. 1993. Phenomenological mapping and comparisons of Shamanic, Buddhist, yogic, and schizophrenic experiences. *Journal of the American Academy of Religion* 61(4): 739–769.
Warner, Richard. 2003. *Recovery from schizophrenia: Psychiatry and political economy*. Psychology Press.
Waxler, N.E. 1974. Culture and mental illness. A social labeling perspective. *The Journal of Nervous and Mental Disease* 159(6): 379–395.
Whitaker, Robert. 2010. *Anatomy of an epidemic: Magic bullets, psychiatric drugs, and the astonishing rise of mental illness in America*, 1st ed. Crown Publishing Group, Division of Random House Inc.

Wittgenstein, Ludwig. 2010. *Philosophical investigations*. New York: Wiley.

Wunderink, L., R.M. Nieboer, D. Wiersma, S. Sytema, and F.J. Nienhuis. 2013. Recovery in remitted first-episode psychosis at 7 years of follow-up of an early dose reduction/discontinuation or maintenance treatment strategy: Long-term follow-up of a 2-year randomized clinical trial. *JAMA Psychiatry* 70(9): 913–920. doi:10.1001/jamapsychiatry.2013.19.

Yang, Lawrence Hsin, Arthur Kleinman, Bruce G. Link, Jo C. Phelan, Sing Lee, and Byron Good. 2007. Culture and stigma: Adding moral experience to stigma theory. *Social Science and Medicine* 64(7): 1524–1535. doi:10.1016/j.socscimed.2006.11.013.

Yanos, P.T., D. Roe, K. Markus, and P.H. Lysaker. 2008. Pathways between internalized stigma and outcomes related to recovery in schizophrenia spectrum disorders. *Psychiatric Services* 59 (12): 1437–1442. doi:10.1176/appi.ps.59.12.1437.

Young, A. 1982. The anthropologies of illness and sickness. *Annual Review of Anthropology* 11 (1): 257–285.

Glossary of Tetum Terms

Bulak A generic but possibly somewhat pejorative term for madness.

Fulan lotuk Both cause and idiom of disordered ("psychotic") speech and behaviour occurring during the new and crescent moon—appears to be associated with, but not identified, as *lulik*.

Hanoin barak Lit. "thinking too much," but colloquially sometimes used as a less pejorative term for *bulak* (madness/psychosis) alongside non-psychotic manifestations of distress.

Lulik Denoting the sacred and by association dangerous and prohibited.

Pontu Generic idiom for madness but which appeared to emphasise the observation of nonsensical speech

Rai nain Powerful spirit of the land (lit. "land lord"), closely related to *lulik*.

J. Rodger and Z. Steel, *Between Trauma and the Sacred*,
Cultural Studies of Science and Medicine, DOI 10.1007/978-3-319-24424-2

Key Author Index

J. Rodger and Z. Steel, *Between Trauma and the Sacred*,
Cultural Studies of Science and Medicine, DOI 10.1007/978-3-319-24424-2

Index

J. Rodger and Z. Steel, *Between Trauma and the Sacred*,
Cultural Studies of Science and Medicine, DOI 10.1007/978-3-319-24424-2

FSC
www.fsc.org
MIX
Papier aus verantwortungsvollen Quellen
Paper from responsible sources
FSC® C105338

If you have any concerns about our products,
you can contact us on
ProductSafety@springernature.com

In case Publisher is established outside the EU,
the EU authorized representative is:
Springer Nature Customer Service Center GmbH
Europaplatz 3, 69115 Heidelberg, Germany

Printed by Libri Plureos GmbH
in Hamburg, Germany